VAGUS NERVE SECRETS EXERCISES AND TECHNIQUES

A SELF-HELP GUIDE TO HELP YOU OVERCOME

ANXIETY AND DEPRESSION.

REAL HELP FOR WEIGHT LOSS, AUTOIMMUNE DISEASES, DIABETES.

© *Copyright 2019 - All rights reserved.*

The content contained within this book may not be reproduced, duplicated or transmitted without direct written permission from the author or the publisher.

Under no circumstances will any blame or legal responsibility be held against the publisher, or author, for any damages, reparation, or monetary loss due to the information contained within this book, either directly or indirectly.

Legal Notice:

This book is copyright protected. It is only for personal use. You cannot amend, distribute, sell, use, quote or paraphrase any part, or the content within this book, without the consent of the author or publisher.

Disclaimer Notice:

Please note the information contained within this document is for educational and entertainment purposes only. All effort has been executed to present accurate, up to date, reliable, complete information. No warranties of any kind are declared or implied. Readers acknowledge that the author is not engaging in the rendering of legal, financial, medical or professional advice. The content within this book has been derived from various sources. Please consult a licensed professional before attempting any techniques outlined in this book.

By reading this document, the reader agrees that under no circumstances is the author responsible for any losses, direct or indirect, that are incurred as a result of the use of information contained within this document, including, but not limited to, errors, omissions, or inaccuracies.

Introduction

Table of Contents

INTRODUCTION 13

CHAPTER 1: UNDERSTANDING THE VAGUS AND ITS MAIN FEATURES 17
- WHAT IS THE VAGUS NERVE? 17
- THE EFFECT OF THE VAGUS NERVE ON YOUR MIND 21
- FEATURES OF THE VAGUS NERVE 22

CHAPTER 2: MAIN FUNCTIONS OF THE VAGUS NERVE 31

THE MIND-BODY CONNECTION 31
- THE VAGUS NERVE AND EMOTIONAL REGULATION 31
- IT HELPS PREVENT INFLAMMATION 32
- GUT-BRAIN COMMUNICATION 34
- CONTROLS OUR BREATHING 34
- VAGUS NERVE AND FEAR 35
- VAGUS NERVE AND MEMORY 35
- OUR NATURAL PACEMAKER 36
- CONTROLS RELAXATION 36
- MONITORS OUR GAG REFLEX 37
- SWEAT CONTROL 38
- STIMULATES PERISTALSIS 38
- CARDIOVASCULAR HEALTH 39
- BREATHING 39

- WEIGHT MANAGEMENT 40
- STRESS MANAGEMENT 40
- IT ASSISTS IN MAKING MEMORIES 41
- IT HELPS IMPROVE YOUR MOOD 41
- GASTROPARESIS 43
- VASOVAGAL SYNCOPE 44
- CHRONIC FATIGUE 45
- IRRITABLE BOWEL SYNDROME 46
- ANXIETY 47
- HEARTBURN 48
- MENTAL HEALTH 48
- CHRONIC INFLAMMATION 49
- BREATHING ISSUES 50
- SENSORY CONDITIONS 51
- DIABETES 51
- HYPERTENSION 52
- ALZHEIMER'S 53
- DEPRESSION 54
- ADRENAL FATIGUE 55
- AUTOIMMUNE VASCULITIS 57
- INFLAMMATORY BOWEL DISEASE 57
- LUPUS 57
- MULTIPLE SCLEROSIS 58
- PSORIASIS 58
- RHEUMATOID ARTHRITIS 58
- MIGRAINES, HEADACHES, AND FIBROMYALGIA 59
- PAIN IN THE EARS 59
- UNUSUAL HEART RATE 60

- DECREASED PRODUCTION OF STOMACH ACID 60
- NAUSEA OR VOMITING 61
- ABDOMINAL BLOATING OR PAIN 61

CHAPTER 4: VAGUS NERVE AND HEALTH CONDITIONS 63
- VAGUS NERVE AND ANXIETY 63
- VAGUS NERVE AND CHRONIC ILLNESS 67
- VAGUS NERVE AND INFLAMMATION 72
- VAGUS NERVE AND PTSD 74
- VAGUS NERVE AND SLEEP DISORDERS 76
- VAGUS NERVE AND GERD 79
- VAGUS NERVE AND HUNGER 82
- BOTOX 86
- CERTAIN ANTIBIOTICS 87
- HEAVY METALS 88
- EXCESSIVE SUGAR 90
- HEALTHY DIET 96
- INTERMITTENT FASTING 108
- PHYSICAL EXERCISE 109
- SLEEP HYGIENE 117
- PROBIOTICS 118
- YOGA AND TAI CHI 120
- MEDITATION 123
- KEEP YOUR STRESS LEVELS IN CHECK 126
- DISEASE MANAGEMENT 127
- WEIGHT MANAGEMENT 127
- GARGLING 128

COFFEE ENEMAS 128
LAUGH LOUD AND LAUGH HARD 132
ELECTRICAL (DIRECT) VAGUS NERVE STIMULATION 133
SINGING TO STIMULATE THE VAGUS NERVE 135
MINDFULNESS TO STIMULATE THE VAGUS NERVE 138
MOVEMENT TO STIMULATE THE VAGUS NERVE 143
SECURITY AND SELF-LOVE 143
GRATITUDE 146
ACUPRESSURE AND ACUPUNCTURE 150
MUSIC AND BINAURAL BEATS 151
PRAYER 153
PRACTICE GENEROSITY 155
CREATE A ROUTINE 157
TIMING: HOW MUCH STIMULATION IS NEEDED? 160

Introduction

Autonomic nervous system a series of nerves within your body that keep you alive. They regulate everything from your heartbeat to your ability to digest food. They control your breathing and ability to manage all of the muscles in your body that are responsible for keeping you alive.

Essentially, your automatic nervous system is responsible for keeping you alive—and it does so entirely unconsciously. You are never aware of the processes in your brain that are actively keeping your heart regulated or your diaphragm moving in regular intervals to keep you alive.

This has one simple function—it allows the brain to communicate with those crucial parts. However, sometimes, that nerve circuit can malfunction, and when it does, there can be significant impacts on the individual.

Just as how a car that has a dysfunctional electrical system may struggle to run effectively, the human body struggles when there are any errors in the vagus nerves.

This book will open your eyes to the myriad of ways that the vagus nerve can directly and negatively impact your life. It is so intrinsically involved in the body's structure that it has even been found to be relevant to treating PTSD, epilepsy, and other chronic diseases. You will be introduced to the importance of the nerve itself before seeing several of the pathologies related to the vagus nerve. Lastly, you will be introduced to several techniques that you can use to stimulate your vagus nerve—in stimulating the vagus nerve, you are able to sort of reset it, allowing yourself to give it the jump-start it needs in order to start working effectively so it can start regulating your body exactly as it was intended to.

As you read through this book, you will learn all of the information that you will need in order to regulate your own vagus nerve with ease—while there are treatments out there that will literally stimulate the vagus nerve for you when implanted, there are also ways that you can essentially trigger your body to regulate it yourself. Ranging from deep breathing to yoga, there are a wide range of ways that you can regulate that nerve, and in doing so, you can find relief.

This book is your guide to becoming more aware of the vagus nerve, finding out how it can help us, and learning more details about it. There is a lot to cover, so let's begin with what the vagus nerve is and dive into its functions. Have you been feeling the effects of stress and anxiety bringing you to an all-time low? Perhaps you have seizures or digestive ailments that just don't seem to right themselves?

Your body is a beautiful piece of work, with so many self-healing methods to get you through the toughest of scenarios. In these pages, we will be diving into the human body to have a look at the Vagus Nerve, and the benefits around its stimulation. We will be touching on how you can use different exercises in order to get you through your highest anxieties, as well as tackling depression and severe illness. Learn how to relax an overstimulated Vagus nerve before it becomes damaged, and spot a damaged nerve with ease. Let's get comfortable, prop up with some pillows, and take an in-depth look into what your system can do for you!

Chapter 1: Understanding the vagus and its main features

What is the Vagus Nerve?

Everything about you is regulated by nerves. From your very thoughts to the way you move your body and what keeps you alive, everything is related to your nerves. Your nerves are the very wiring that allows you to exist and function. They are the wiring that connects the body to the mind and they run throughout the whole body. They are different sizes, all running to different areas, and allowing your entire body to interact as once integrated being, one complete system that is entirely able to work together effectively and cohesively.

Nerves themselves are cells that allow for electrochemical nerve impulses to travel throughout the body. These impulses, known as action potentials, are how the nerves communicate with each other. When you touch or otherwise interact with something, nerves have activated that trigger and send those same action potentials back throughout the nervous system and all the way to the brain, where they are then processed and treated accordingly.

These nerves are formed by an axon, which processes the impulse, and the sheathing around it. The nerves are said to innervate or provide information and control, certain parts of the body. When an area is innervated by a specific nerve, that means that the particular nerve being discussed is responsible for the sensory movement and information at that spot.

Your nerves are designed to carry impulses and action potentials almost instantaneously—they may trigger immediately and some of the fastest nerves are able to process at a speed of 120 m/s, during which the impulse is constantly being translated from an electrical impulse into a chemical impulse at the end of the axon, where chemicals are then released that interact with the next nerve in line in the sequence, where the nerve is then triggered, cuing it to create another electrical impulse.

These particular nerves are known to have sensory functions, whereas some of the other cranial nerves within your body will have more control over your movements and well as controlling certain muscles and gland functions. These are better known as motor functions.

The vagus nerve is an anomaly all on its own. This particular nerve has both sensory and motor functions, while most other cranial nerves will only have one or the other of these functions. The vagus nerve itself, you will find, somehow keeps track of way more than we realize.

The vagus nerve will also have an almost reverse effect too, where not only is it delivering information from the brain to each of these organs, but it is also sending signals from the organs to go back to the brain to react accordingly. In order for this to happen, the vagus nerve contains two separate bunches of nerve cells that are connecting the organs and body to the brain stem.

These cells allow the brain to receive information from the organs relating to their different functions, and can therefore monitor what is happening within our bodies, should the need arise to fix something that has gone faulty.

Your vagus nerve helps control movement and sensory information for the heart, lungs, abdomen, and the neck, but it performs several functions in the body. However, in order to understand the functions, you need to understand something about the nervous system.

Your nervous system works in two areas, parasympathetic and sympathetic. The sympathetic part of the nervous system is responsible for boosting your heart and breathing rate, blood pressure, energy levels and how alert you are. You don't need to think about this side of things, since it is all automatic.

There have even been connections made between the types of food eaten and how the vagus nerve reacts. It can end up irritated and inflamed due to eating spicy food or alcohol. You can even end up with an inflamed vagus nerve when you're stressed out or anxious . . . which in turn can cause stress and anxiety.

It's all connected and the vagus nerve is the center of it all. When you manage your vagus nerve and keep it in good condition, your body parts will work in unison.

That's the end goal, to ensure that your entire body is working, rather than treating just one part that is causing problems. Unfortunately, that's exactly what many doctors do, treat the individual problem. However, if one of your organs is not working properly, that is going to affect more organs and it's best to look at everything as a whole.

The effect of the Vagus Nerve on Your Mind

The vagus nerve can have an effect on your memories and thought processes. It's been linked to hormone production that stimulates the fight or flight response, feelings of happiness or contentment, and the lack of these can result in an imbalance within the brain. Anxiety, depression, and other mental health issues are all affected by the vagus nerve and whether it tells the brain to produce the necessary hormones or not.

Stimulation of the nerve has proven useful in a variety of ways. Not only can a functioning vagus nerve help prevent issues like depression or anxiety, it can also be useful in building memories. If you need to remember things better or plan to study for an exam, it can actually help if you stimulate the vagus nerve. You'll remember better and it improves neuroplasticity or the ability to learn. In fact, it's even been shown to help with conditions like dementia and Alzheimer's.

Features of the Vagus Nerve

One of the greatest anomalies about the vagus nerve is that it is the major parasympathetic nerve of the entire body! The vagus nerve is in charge of many of the body's main functions that all seem a bit strange to be linked together. Have you noticed that when you clean your ears out and stimulate the ear canal, you cough? That is because the cough reflex is directly linked to ear canal stimulation.

The vagus nerve is also directly linked to your gag reflex when the back and sides of the throat are stimulated, it is linked to slowing your heart rate, and it can control your sweating and regulate your blood pressure. It can also stimulate peristalsis of the gastrointestinal tract as well as being able to control your vascular tone.

The vagus nerve has both sensory as well as motor functions that keep us ticking the way we should. Some of these functions include:

- The stimulation of muscles in the soft palate, which is in the roof of your mouth, as well as stimulating the larynx and pharynx inside your throat.

- Heart stimulation, which thereafter helps to lower your heart rate as well as regulate your blood pressure.
- The stimulation of the digestive tract in order to help you with digestion and passing your food through your system. This also includes stimulation of the esophagus.
- Stimulation of the sensitive skin behind your ears as a sensory piece, as well as sending information to the brain to trigger reflexes when stimulation is affecting the outer ear canal as well as the throat. You will also find that it plays a part in your taste sensations at the back of your mouth where the root of your tongue is.

When the vagus nerve gets stimulated very suddenly without any warning, you can cause a reaction called the vasovagal reflex to happen. When you get a vasovagal reflex, you often find that it causes a sudden drop in blood pressure as well as your heart rate will slow down dramatically.

There are some people who are unfortunately prone to getting these reflexes although it is most commonly found due to stress, high amounts of pain, getting a sudden fright or even from a gastrointestinal problem from something you may have eaten that didn't quite agree with your insides.

Considering it is in charge of some of the most important functions within your body, namely regulating your ability to have a beating heart and breathe, it becomes incredibly apparent that your vagus nerve is incredibly important. In fact, it is believed to be one of the most important nerves within the body. Without it, or with it completely dysfunctional, a normal existence would be nearly impossible. Because of the fact that it is so crucial to so many of these important functions to survive, it has garnered plenty of attention in recent days.

Without the vagus nerve, you will be unable to do anything. You could not digest your food. You could not breathe when you slept. Your heart would stop beating. You would cease to live. The vagus nerve, when dysfunctional, disrupts nearly every major function in some way—it can lead to heart irregularities, breathing irregularities, digestive problems, and more, all because without this simple nerve pair, the brain cannot regulate it. Largely speaking, the importance of the vagus nerve lies in the fact that it is directly influential to the regulation of the autonomic nervous system.

This nerve becomes incredibly crucial to understand for one crucial reason—you can regulate it with ease. You can use the vagus nerve, learning how to stimulate it when necessary to regulate your own body. The nerve is there, just waiting for you to truly utilize it, and if you do, you are able to regulate the response of it simply by knowing how to regulate yourself.

When this vasovagal reflex does happen, it will cause your heart rate and blood pressure to drop very quickly, most often causing loss of consciousness or fainting. This is a condition that is called vasovagal syncope.

When the vagus nerve gets stimulated for therapeutic effects, you will find that you are able to have complete control over your body!

You can stimulate the vagus nerve to stop a nasty hiccup episode that is relentless, and doctors will often use the vagus nerve to help them diagnose a potential heart murmur or to treat depression.

In order for your brain to know the current status of what is happening to the organs around your body, it needs the signals from the vagus nerve to bounce back through those organs and send a sort of 'report' back to the brain in order to react further.

The vagus nerve has become so important in the medical industry that doctors are now finding that they can stimulate the vagus nerve using a device that gets placed in your chest, somewhat like a pacemaker, and send signals to the nerve through this device in order to get certain reactions from your body. Vagus nerve blocking is also fast becoming a popular method of treatment, especially aiding in weight loss as it has become far more superior to that of gastric bypass surgery!

The vagus nerve also serves a very interesting purpose when it comes to the flight or fight mode that our bodies go into when something is wrong. Stimulation of the vagus nerve can result in relaxation after a situation that has left us feeling overly stressed or trapped in that fight or flight mode.

It will also indicate to us when we are in potential danger and need to keep our guard up and our wits about us, keeping us safe in the long run like an animal's instincts would. During emotional stress, if the vagus nerve is overstimulated, it can overcompensate for the sympathetic nervous system and ultimately cause a vasovagal syncope as your heart rate can suddenly drop. It is said that vasovagal syncope is more likely to affect women and children than it does men, and can often lead to loss of bladder control in the moments leading up to an extreme fear or stressful situation.

Because the vagus nerve has efferent fibers that pass through the pharynx as well as the back of your throat, it therefore becomes responsible for your gag reflex, as well as having these nerve endings going straight down the esophagus. The stimulation of these receptors can potentially cause vomiting and in the long run, if overstimulated, may also result in a vasovagal response as discussed earlier.

Our brain does not just react to external stimuli to keep our environment safe and conducive for us, it also requires constant communication with other body organs. Communication between the brain and other body organs serves to ensure the optimal functioning of the various body systems is maintained. Body organs require regulation such that processes can be activated or inhibited depending on the situation or physical state of our bodies.

If, for instance, you are jogging, your body will require more oxygen to facilitate the increased demand that is occasioned by physical activity. For this to happen, the heart and breathing rates need to increase, so that more air is pumped by the lungs and blood circulation is enhanced to increase the supply of this oxygen to the tissues and muscles. This ability of the body to regulate functions and maintain homeostasis is crucial for normal function and our overall health and wellbeing.

Without the effective functioning of the vagus nerve, the sympathetic nervous becomes overstimulated, and this, in turn, causes organ malfunction. To ensure that our vagal tone is high, there are measures we can take to routinely activate its parasympathetic effects and ensure that we reap the benefits of its self-healing power. We can activate the vagus nerve using various techniques such as meditation, exercise, breathing techniques, cold therapy, and many other techniques.

Chapter 2: Main functions of the Vagus Nerve

The Mind-Body Connection

The mind and body are closely interrelated—two sides to the same coin, and yet, they cannot fully communicate without help. The nerves, namely the vagus nerve, communicates between the two, creating the conduit through which the nerve impulses are translated and passed along to enable the body to communicate with the brain. Without these impulses, the nervous system cannot get the regulation it needs. The mind cannot regulate the body if it does not receive feedback from the body. The vagus nerve allows for that input, and then it allows you to regulate the body as well. Because the vagus nerve is so closely related to awareness and keeping the human body alive and processing, it is crucial to human survival.

The Vagus Nerve and Emotional Regulation

Another crucial factor of the vagus nerve is the fact that it is directly responsible for your ability to self-regulate. It is what calms you when you are stressed. When you meditate or do yoga to relax or calm yourself, you are unknowingly activating your vagus nerve. That stimulation creates the calming effect that you are feeling.

That emotional regulation is powerful. It means that people can take control of their emotional states with a deep breathing exercise or some other method that will allow for a trigger and stimulation of the vagus nerve. When you learn this process, you give yourself another coping mechanism, a way to relieve your suffering and take your own mental wellness into your own hands. If you are afraid? You are able to activate your vagus nerve to help. Suffering from PTSD? Your vagus nerve can help with that, too.

Several issues can be managed relatively simply, all through learning to take control of your vagus nerve.

It Helps Prevent Inflammation

Inflammation is just one step in the process of healing. When your body is attacked by external forces, such as toxins, injuries, and infections that enter the body through openings or damages to the skin, then inflammation is a way for the body to fight against those forces. The body activates it when something damages or attacks your cells. It begins the process of inflammation by first releasing chemicals that encourage the immune system to respond.

The entire process of inflammation usually lasts anywhere from a few hours to a few days. In such cases, we usually refer to the process as acute inflammation.

The state of stress is called chronic inflammation and it creates all kinds of trouble to the body, down to the organs and the tissues. Inflammation can be treated with the vagus nerve. It can also prevent inflammation as well. When you get injured, whether it be a cut, scrape, or anything else, you will notice some redness on the surface of your skin. This is totally normal.

The vagus nerve is able to effectively control inflammation by inhibiting the overstimulation of the immune system that is caused by the sympathetic nervous system. Medical research has shown that stimulation of the vagus nerve helps in resolving conditions related to prolonged inflammation of tissues in the body.

Gut-Brain Communication

The vagus nerve is also where the brain and the gut communicate with one another. For example, if you ate something that didn't taste good, your vagus nerve will send a signal to the brain telling it that you don't want to eat whatever it was. Sometimes, if you're anxious about something, that funny feeling you get in your stomach is attributed to the nerve. Your vagus nerve is responsible for all that communication.

Controls Our Breathing

Breathing is a big part of our lives. The purpose of breathing isn't just simply to take in air; it's also important because it helps bring oxygen to our organs. Without oxygen, and without supplying our vital organs with it, we risk not being alive. However, sometimes breathing into much air can end up hurting us later on. You've probably been in a situation where you take in short but quick breaths of air; this often happens when you're anxious or nervous.

The vagus nerve also helps with relaxation. After a long day, I'm sure the first thing you want to do is sit on your couch and relax. The vagus nerve sends a signal to your body telling it that it wants to relax. As a result, the vagus nerve will also communicate to your diaphragm; the diaphragm will expand, thereby allowing more air into your system. This will help you feel more relaxed as you're able to take in longer and deeper breaths.

Vagus Nerve And Fear

Fear is something we all experience at some point. If we've ever been in a situation where we've felt fearful, the vagus nerve is at play in those cases. When you feel scared, your vagus nerve will send that information straight to the brain. Your brain will then accept the signal sent from the vagus nerve and warn you. As a result, your fight or flight response is triggered.

Vagus Nerve And Memory

When you recall something, you release the neurotransmitter called norepinephrine deep into the amygdala, which is where our memories are stored. This could also account for why you experience an uncomfortable gut feeling when you're afraid, because the vagus nerve records the information of how you feel when scared and can recognize when you are scared again.

Our Natural Pacemaker

While we already discussed that the vagus nerve controls our heart and blood pressure, it also serves as a natural pacemaker.

If you've never heard of a pacemaker before, or have never seen one, it's essentially a small device placed near your heart which sends out electrical signals directly to the heart to help it push out impulses. However, we already have a natural pacemaker in our bodies; therefore, not necessarily needing additional devices. You can measure your heart rate by keeping track of the number of beats. This will show your heart rate variability. The vagus nerve takes this information and then determines whether or not it needs to encourage the heart to pump more blood. So, the vagus nerve doesn't just help your heart rate but it also provides the heart with all the necessary information it needs to work its magic.

Controls Relaxation

Your vagus nerve is responsible for pumping out acetylcholine, which is the hormone that tells your body to relax. The sympathetic nervous system pumps out cortisol and adrenaline, while the vagus nerve does the opposite.

What's amazing about this is that it can tell so many parts of your body to relax when it's experiencing high levels of stress. Imagine the vagus nerve as a control center, whereby it is in control of all the different parts of the body. It sends out signals to different areas of the body whenever enzymes or proteins need to be released. Some of the different chemicals your vagus nerve secretes include vasopressin, which helps with water loss; oxytocin, which helps with pain relief; and prolactin, which helps with milk secretion and promotes sexual potency. The vagus nerve controls a lot of the hormones within the body, hence why it's so important for us.

Monitors Our Gag Reflex

Your gag reflex is also stimulated by the vagus nerve. If something is going down the wrong pipe, your vagus nerve will immediately stimulate your gag reflex, causing you likely to cough. This cough reflex can also be stimulated through our ear canal. When there's something that shouldn't be in the ear canal, chances are your cough reflex will react and you will be forced to cough. These reflexes also ensure that your body is safe and secure, free of anything harmful.

Sweat Control

The vagus nerve also controls sweat, or lack thereof. When the body gets too hot, your vagus nerve will tell the body to secrete sweat to help cool it down. You may also experience excessive sweating whenever you're scared. Sometimes, sweating is a sign that you probably should leave the situation you're currently in. The vagus nerve, while also controlling your heart rate and your hormones, is also important for stimulation of the sweat glands in your body.

Stimulates Peristalsis

In essence, it's a slow, pulsating motion which pushes contents. This is also where the vagus nerve can stimulate the gallbladder to form bile. Bile is produced from the broken down food. Peristalsis is something that happens in the digestive tract. If peristalsis does not function the way it's supposed to, or if you experience trouble with your bowels, this might be the cause of the food you ate and how it was digested. There are a few different types of disorders that this can cause if the vagus nerve isn't properly stimulated, but we'll get into those later.

The vagus nerve is responsible for a lot of different things that can happen in the body; therefore, when you're looking to improve the health of the vagus nerve, these various functions should all be considered, and understanding their functions is just as important.

Cardiovascular Health

The vagus nerve functions in the control of our heart rate, in effect, acting as a natural pacemaker. By stimulating heart muscles, it can effectively slow down our heart rate when it is too fast as happens in stressful conditions.

Breathing

Our ability to breathe is controlled by our lungs, which are regulated by the Vagus nerve through the neurotransmitter acetylcholine. Proper breathing is not only an effective way to deal with pain but is also effective in coping with stress by creating a calming effect on the body. Relaxation techniques such as meditation and yoga incorporate breathing techniques because proper breathing has a relaxing effect on the body.

Weight management

When the vagus nerve cannot send a message to the brain that the stomach is full, it means you will not be able to know when you are full or not, and this is likely to cause overeating.

Stimulating the vagus nerve increases its sensitivity to the fullness signal from the stomach, and this increased sensitivity will cause you to feel fuller faster and, as such, will result in reduced food intake.

Stress management

When the body's sympathetic responses have been activated, we go into flight and fight mode.

However, when cortisol levels remain elevated for prolonged periods of time, it has a myriad of harmful effects, including weight gain, high blood pressure, insomnia, and chronic fatigue. The vagus nerve, with its parasympathetic effects of inhibiting sympathetic responses, can effectively inhibit the release of cortisol by putting your body back into a rested and relaxed state. It is for this reason that people with a stronger vagus nerve response recover faster from illness or stress.

It Assists in Making Memories

Most people think that memories are only confined to a certain area or a few areas of the brain. It's like how we place wardrobes in our homes; you don't usually find one in the kitchen and one in the bathroom for good measure. They are stored in certain areas and they contain your clothing and valuables. However, memories are also related to the connections between neurons. In other words, a particular pattern in the neural network of your brain activates a certain memory.

It Helps Improve Your Mood

Your thyroid, adrenal and sex hormones all come together to help you with your mood. They release chemicals that cause an imbalance in your system. For example, your thyroid hormones are released from a specific gland located in your neck. These hormones are important and they not only manage metabolism and your body temperature, but they also play a vital part in your brain chemistry, too.

Chapter 3: Vagus Nerve inflamed or altered: Body Symptoms

The effect of the vagus nerve on the heart rate, breathing, and digestive function means that it is important to have this nerve functioning at optimum levels if we are to maintain proper organ function as well as optimum mental health. Some of the symptoms that can be associated with poor functioning of the vagus nerve include:

Gastroparesis

This condition affects the ability of the stomach to empty itself by affecting the contractions that move food along the digestive tract. This condition can result in bloating, blood sugar fluctuations, vomiting, loss of appetite, or abdominal pain. One of the first issues is a condition called gastroparesis and is a sign of a damaged vagus nerve.

Gastroparesis is a condition where the stomach isn't able to empty itself in the ways that it should. When this occurs, nausea, heartburn, the feeling of fullness, and vomiting may occur.

But, if you are experiencing gastroparesis, there are no contractions, which causes a lot of problems, including nausea and vomiting. The nausea you get from gastroparesis can lead to vomiting of food that has not yet been digested.

Your appetite will be affected too. You may either not want to eat, or if you try to eat, you'll only be able to take in a little bit of food, simply because you'll instantly feel full. Sometimes, this will in turn cause a lot of weight loss.

Gastroparesis also affects the bloating of the body. Most people who have a vagus nerve that's not working properly will experience bloating, or have severe abdominal pain.

Vasovagal syncope

Vasovagal syncope is a common condition that is associated with the heart. Vasovagal syncope can cause your heart rate as well as blood pressure to suddenly drop to levels that are below normal, thereby causing an individual to faint.

Since the vagus nerve is widely spread out through the body with sensory and motor effects on various tissues in the body, when it ceases to function properly, there is undoubtedly a myriad of symptoms that arise. The symptoms that will manifest will be dependent on part or section of the vagus nerve that is affected. If you don't care for the vagus nerve, you may notice some significant changes with your heart health. Chances are, if your vagus nerve isn't working properly, you will experience a rapid heart rate or a slow one. Bradycardia is the term used to refer to a slower than normal heart rate. Opposite of this is tachycardia, which is the result of a more than normal increased heart rate. In some cases, tachycardia can actually make your heart beat more than 100 times a minute, which isn't healthy for the muscle, and can cause it to overwork the body. Either one of these conditions can lead to other issues with your heart and other vital organs in the body.

Chronic fatigue

Fatigue is the feeling of exhaustion, both physically and mentally and is usually characterized by an overall lack of motivation and energy. While it is ordinary to feel weary after a long day at the office or intense physical activity, chronic fatigue is characterized by a lack of energy and feeling of general malaise that cannot be attributed to one particular cause.

If you are suffering from chronic fatigue, you will find that you tend to feel tired, even first thing in the morning, just after waking up. You experience a sluggish feeling that stays with you throughout the day, and you may even be prone to feeling you do not want to do anything at all. If you find yourself constantly feeling tired, with little energy, and no motivation to face the day even when you have just woken up, you might need to check the health of your vagus nerve. Infection of the vagus can lead to an individual developing chronic fatigue.

Irritable bowel syndrome

The vagus nerve plays a significant role in enabling digestive functions, and when it is not working properly, abdominal disorders become a possible symptom. The inflammation of the cells lining the digestive tract due to prolonged fight or flight response activation can lead to bowel irritation.

When the vagus nerve is doing its job properly, it mitigates inflammation by inhibiting sympathetic responses. However, when the vagus nerve is malfunctioning, the sympathetic responses become prolonged, leading to inflammation.

Anxiety

Life is full of ups and downs. From work-related pressure, relationship problems, and family dysfunction, there are multiple experiences and situations that cause anxiety to the ordinary person. In most cases, you should be able to deal with anxiety as it comes and goes.

Stresses activate our sympathetic responses, which equip us for flight or fight by priming our bodies for action. For your body to revert to a rested state from this state of agitation, the vagus nerve parasympathetic responses need to override the responses initiated by the sympathetic nervous system.

This means the vagus nerve should be able to slow down your heart rate and breathing rate so that you can feel calm and relaxed. If this parasympathetic mechanism of the vagus nerve does not work properly, you will be prone to chronic anxiety which, in turn, can result in chronic inflammation or even depression.

Heartburn

The hypersensitivity to acid reflux is referred to as heartburn. We have all, at some point, experienced that burning feeling in our throats after eating certain kinds of food. This burning sensation is typically our body's response to excessive acid in the digestive tract.

The vagus nerve plays a vital role in the communication between the gut and brain, and if this communication pathway is disrupted, the regulation of the gut can be impaired, which can result in the accumulation of acid and heartburn as a result.

Mental Health

The vagus nerve, and not taking proper care of it, can cause you to experience an array of mental health issues. Remember, your emotions are connected to how you feel; therefore, if you're constantly feeling tired, have no appetite, cannot think positively, chances are you're likely experiencing a mental health condition such as depression or anxiety.

The vagus nerve plays a huge role in how your mental health is affected. If you're constantly feeling tired, sad, or anxious, your vagus nerve is a likely cause of this. It's important that you don't ignore the signs; identifying them early on can lead you back on the right path.

Chronic Inflammation

Chronic inflammation and fatigue are also two things that happen as a result of a vagus nerve being out of sorts.

Remember, when your vagus nerve isn't working properly, it can't step in to fix issues with pain, inflammation, etc. Therefore, a vagus nerve that isn't working properly can't identify when you're experiencing inflammation and fix the problem. This will lead you to experience chronic inflammation, meaning you'll have inflammation for longer periods of time.

Some of the most common conditions and diseases that are linked to chronic inflammation include arthritis, asthma, ulcers (including peptic ulcers), Crohn's disease, sinusitis, hepatitis, and type one diabetes. If you notice any signs of abnormal inflammation, or chronic inflammation, see a specialist as soon as possible. It's possible that you develop one of the conditions or diseases listed above.

Autoimmune diseases are also another issue. Autoimmune diseases may not be noticeable on the surface, but they will be felt internally.

As a result, you'll no doubt feel more tired and constantly fatigued. Autoimmune diseases can occur when your parasympathetic nervous system is at its lowest, therefore causing those feelings of fatigue.

Breathing Issues

Breathing issues are another result of your vagus nerve not being taken care of. The vagus nerve is responsible for regulating your breathing as well as the fibers that move through the respiratory tract. When people have an overstimulated vagus nerve, oftentimes, they experience shortness of breath or an inability to get the most out of your breathing. This can cause some to faint, feel numbness, and overall have difficulty breathing; neither is a pleasant experience to say the least. It may cause you to develop respiratory issues. The longer your vagus nerve remains overstimulated, the more problems it may cause in the future. Ensuring that it's working as it should will also help ensure that you never endure any issues with breathing.

Sensory Conditions

Sensory conditions may develop if your vagus nerve is not taken care of. Specifically, the ability to listen, and to taste certain foods and such. The vagus nerve is responsible for the sensors that you have in your palate and epiglottis, which are in charge of your ability to taste. An uncared for vagus nerve may cause you to lose your ability to taste certain foods or liquids. Your tongue may not be able to handle certain types of food, causing you to potentially develop other conditions related to eating. You may also experience greater levels of nausea, and sometimes even vomiting.

Diabetes

The primary source of energy in the body for cellular functions is blood glucose. When we consume food, glucose is extracted from the food and then broken down in the presence of the hormone insulin to generate energy for various cell functions. The hormone insulin is a necessary component in the breakdown of glucose.

In situations where we have developed low insulin levels or insulin insensitivity, cells are, as a result, unable to access energy from glucose in the blood. This results in hyperglycemia or the presence of excess glucose in the blood, which is brought about by the lack of efficient breakdown of glucose.

Hypertension

The force that your blood exerts on blood vessels is referred to as blood pressure. Hypertension refers to a state in which the blood pressure is elevated higher than what is ideal for good health. High blood pressure can cause a myriad of complications such as stroke, heart diseases, or even kidney failure. It is, therefore, important to ensure that we effectively manage our blood pressure to avoid health complications that may be fatal.

Chronic stress is a major predisposing factor for hypertension. The vagus nerve has a significant impact on stress management, meaning it is equally effective in regulating blood pressure and reducing the chances of hypertension. When our fight or flight responses are activated by the sympathetic nervous system to enable us to deal with emotional or physical stresses, our vital organs are strained by the increased demand for energy in the body. In this stressed state, our heart rate increases, our rate of respiration equally goes up, and our digestive tract functions are inhibited.

Chronic Stress

Conflicts, work-related pressure, bills, dysfunction in family or relationships, illness, and so many more factors have made the levels of stress to rise significantly in recent years. Life is challenging in more ways than one, and as a result, stress has become a common part of our existence and daily life.

What most people do not know is that our body responds to both physical and emotional or perceived stress in the same way. This means that a hiker facing a physical threat from a mountain lion and someone having a panic attack because they are afraid of giving a public speech will elicit the same physiological reactions in the body. In both cases, the sympathetic responses of fight or flight will be initiated.

Alzheimer's

Alzheimer's is a cognitive disorder characterized by loss of memory, impairment of the ability to think clearly, and the progressive loss of behavioral and social engagement skills. This disorder results from the gradual degeneration and death of brain cells, which, in turn, causes the impairment of brain functions and cognitive abilities.

Alzheimer's ultimately leads to dementia which is a condition referencing the decline in mental function that results in an individual being unable to live and function normally. Alzheimer's presents as a progressive ailment starting with forgetfulness and memory loss and progressing to an inability to perform even simple and straightforward tasks.

Depression

Depression is a severe mental disorder that can affect how you feel act and think. Until recently, depression was considered to be just a person experiencing a bad mood or passing anxiety. In actual sense, depression is much more than just feeling low or being in a bad mood. It is a mental state that is characterized by emotional detachment, feelings of sadness or loss, and a lack of interest in activities. Depression is a serious mental illness that has been linked to suicide and destructive social behavior.

Is it possible to determine the cause of depression? While it is not possible to single out a single factor as the main course of depression, social factors, biological, and psychological sources of distress have been found to be predisposing factors that lead to depressive tendencies. This distress that is initiated by a combination of these factors alters and impairs brain function resulting in psychological and even physical disorders.

Depression weakens your immune system leaving you susceptible to infections that your body could easily ward off if you were not depressed. It has also been associated with poor weight management. Have you ever noticed that you tend to either eat too much when you are feeling low or to not eat at all? Depression has an undeniable effect on our weight by causing us to become obese through overeating or underweight by not eating enough. While binge eating after you have had a stressful day will probably not have long term effects on your health, people with chronic depression develop long-term bad eating habits, which ultimately impact their health.

Adrenal fatigue

When the vagus nerve is either overworking or not working enough, the hypothalamus stops signaling the pituitary gland appropriately, which results in overproduction of some hormones and not enough of others.

The net effect of this hormonal imbalance that is created in the body is that every problem either starts to feel like the end of the world, or you find yourself not acknowledging real issues that need to be addressed.

These extremes that are triggered by hormonal imbalance can lead to disorders such as insomnia, lack of motivation, anxiety, chronic stress, and fatigue. This condition where the adrenal glands are not able to respond appropriately to stimuli is referred to as adrenal fatigue.

Vagus nerve stimulation can help in keeping your hormonal balance in check and reduce the tendency to get worked up or stressed over small issues that can be resolved.

Autoimmune vasculitis

When the immune system attacks blood vessels, it can cause serious issues. The resulting inflammation actually squeezes the arteries and veins, nearly closing them and preventing proper circulation. This causes some pretty obvious health risks that should be avoided.

Inflammatory bowel disease

Commonly known as IBD, there are a few sub-diseases under this. It refers to inflammation of the intestinal walls, but depending on where it is, the disease has a specific name.

Lupus

Systemic lupus erythematosus is another autoimmune disease that you have probably heard of. Originally thought to be a skin issue, it has now become evident that lupus affects many internal organs as well.

Most commonly, the immune system attacks the brain, kidneys, joints, and the heart, causing pain and fatigue.

Multiple sclerosis

MS is one of the more deadly autoimmune diseases. In this case, the nervous system is attacked and the protective myelin around the nerves is destroyed. This results in poor communication between the body and brain, which makes people feel numb and gradually lose the ability to walk and balance. It slowly robs the affected person of their ability to move and do things on their own, even affecting speech, until eventually it affects even heart and lung function.

Psoriasis

Everyone grows new skin cells on a regular basis and we are constantly losing or shedding old skin cells. With psoriasis, the immune system attacks the skin and causes the cells to grow far too fast. They build up in patches and become inflamed and itchy. Psoriasis can also pass to the joints and cause a form of arthritis that is very painful.

Rheumatoid arthritis

This form of autoimmune disease involves the joints. Your immune system goes after the joints and you'll find that your joints tend to be hot, red, and stiff. It can be so painful as to affect your daily activities.

Migraines, Headaches, and Fibromyalgia

Pain is one of the things that nerves transmit very well, sometimes too well, and in this chapter, we'll focus on some of the more common types of pain. The pains caused in this section tend to be the result of an oversensitive pain transmission system, which means the vagus nerve is transmitting extreme pain where there should likely only be a minor amount.

Pain in the ears

The ears are very closely related to your vagus nerve as we saw in the previous chapter. If you are experiencing pain in an ear, it could just be from a minor infection, although it could also very well be from the vagus nerve wreaking havoc with your system. If you see a healthcare provider for your ear ache, they will be able to shine a light into the ear canal in order to check if there is anything wrong with the inner, middle, or outer ear itself, or whether it could be that your vagus nerve is damaged and is the cause for the pain.

Unusual heart rate

If your heart is currently either going way too fast without having run a marathon in the Olympics, or even if it seems to be unreasonably slow, it may indicate that the vagus nerve has been affected and is causing either the sympathetic or parasympathetic nervous system to work overtime. This is a very serious symptom and should be dealt with immediately by a doctor or healthcare practitioner. Delaying the process of seeking help can potentially be fatal, so get it sorted sooner rather than later.

Decreased production of stomach acid

Naturally, if the vagus nerve isn't in optimal condition, neither is your digestive system. This means that you will also have decreased production of stomach acid, leading to a rather painful system when it comes down to bowel movements. This will also prevent your body from soaking in any vital nutrients through the intestines and stomach lining and what goes in, will most likely come out in the exact same fashion.

Nausea or vomiting

Nausea and vomiting are also closely related to how the stomach reacts when the vagus nerve is under stress or damaged in any way. If there is damage to the vagus nerve, the body sees this as an illness and will most of the time try to purge out what may be causing the problem. Thus, even though the problem itself is nothing that you may have eaten or ingested, your stomach may still react by releasing bile into the intestines causing mild to severe nausea and vomiting.

Abdominal bloating or pain

When the vagus nerve is under attack, you may experience excessive abdominal pain or possibly bloating due to the nerves that are directly connected to the intestines and digestive system.

Chapter 4: Vagus Nerve And Health Conditions

Vagus Nerve and Anxiety

Anxiety itself is one of the most common mental health issues in the world. While anxiety on its own is sometimes normal, healthy, and totally expected, such as if you are going to your first day at a new job, or if you have a job interview, it is important to understand that if your anxiety has become such a constant in your life that you are always struggling, always suffering, and always attempting to get out from underneath that stress, it could be a problem in your life.

When you are anxious, your fear drive is on auto-pilot. You may feel a sense of dread deep within yourself that you cannot explain or regulate. You may feel like you have no way to stop those feelings of fear and dread, and oftentimes, it can be incredibly difficult to do so if you are not armed and prepared. Sometimes, it could be a dull pang, a quiet whisper in the back of your mind telling you that you are not good enough, but other times, it can be so extreme, so detrimental, that you find yourself legitimately panicking for no reason. It can manifest as phobias, as obsessions and compulsions, or as panic attacks. Other times, it can manifest as just a deep-seated feeling of dread and terror. Nevertheless, it is important to recognize just how that anxiety can impact your life.

Beyond that, however, the longer the sympathetic nervous system is allowed to rule, the more stressed and anxious the body becomes, creating higher levels of cortisol and glutamate, both of which stress out the body even further. This means that you are left feeling miserable.

The vagus nerve, of course, is going to be sending impulses back to your brain to fill it in with how the body is feeling, due to its afferent status. The longer this stress goes on as well, the less likely it is that the parasympathetic nervous system will kick into play in the first place, meaning that you will be less likely to be able to defeat that anxiety at any given point in time. Unless you are able to kick-start your vagus nerve back in gear to get it moving, you are going to struggle.

Vagus Nerve and Depression

Depression is characterized by the negative feelings associated with it. Those suffering from depression at any point in time feel as though they are sad or hopeless much of the time. They may struggle to find interest, value, or purpose in most things that they are doing at any given point in time, and because of that, they struggle to function.

As they grow more and more depressed, they struggle further and further with interacting with other people. They cannot manage the life that they once did, feeling as though their ability to focus has gone away, and even if they could focus, they would find little use in doing so in the first place.

Depression itself comes in many different shapes and forms, ranging from major depressive episodes to seasonal affective disorder. Each of these can have their own impacts on one's life, however, and even mild depression is just as worthy of treatment as major depressive disorders.

In order to be diagnosed with depression, the symptoms of depression must be persistent and consistent, lasting at least 2 weeks in which symptoms are severe. Those with more mild depression are oftentimes likely to take much longer for diagnosis than those who have severe depressive disorder.

Despite the fact that depression seems to hit women twice as often as men, possibly due to hormone fluctuations related to the menstrual cycle and pregnancies of women, anyone can suffer from depression. Adult or child, man or women, anyone can potentially suffer, and when they are left without treatment, it could last for months or years.

Despite the fact that most forms of depression can be treated with less invasive methods, the fact that vagus nerve stimulation can treat depression implies that there is some involvement there. While it is not entirely known why stimulating the vagus nerve will trigger an improvement in depression, especially treatment resistant depression that has been difficult to treat in the first place, it has been found to be effective.

That inflammation in particular could potentially be related to depression. It has been found that those with this increase in inflammation can lead to the depressed mood. The inflammation lessens serotonin levels within the brain, which then leads to mood regulation problems. After all, depression is commonly treated with selective serotonin reuptake inhibitors (SSRIs), which create larger concentrations of serotonin in the brain to combat the symptoms altogether.

The implication, then, is that the lack of stimulation from the vagus nerve allows the sympathetic nervous system to run rampant. That causes an inflammatory response within the body, which then also creates the response in which the body struggles to produce enough serotonin. That lack of serotonin, then, is linked to the depressive symptoms.

Vagus Nerve and Chronic Illness

Chronic illnesses are relatively vague—there are several entirely unrelated diseases and conditions that could be considered chronic. In order to be considered chronic, there are a few criteria that must be met: the condition must be long-lasting, require medical care, and/or it may limit daily activities and functioning.

These illnesses and diseases, despite the fact that they are long-lasting and limiting, are still not always fatal. Chronic illnesses are largely considered to be manageable, and while they absolutely do directly impact your quality of life, they do not necessarily condemn you to an early death. You can live an entire, mostly whole, life with a chronic illness that is being effectively managed by a medical professional with a treatment plan that works for you.

Effectively, chronic illnesses are usually considered to be illnesses or conditions that are long-lasting. Despite the fact that they sometimes come with remission stages, in which the sufferer remains relatively symptom free, people usually see a relapse after which the symptoms return. These illnesses can be contagious or entirely non-communicable, depending on the condition in particular.

Often, when you see "chronic condition" used to describe something, it is usually describing some sort of syndrome, any sort of impairment, a disability, or a disease. So long as it meets the criteria, it will be considered a chronic condition.

Chronic illnesses and conditions, like the people who suffer from them, come in a wide variety of shapes and sizes. These can include anything from cancer to HIV, with nearly everything in between considered a chronic ailment.

Some of these can be problems with pain while others can mental health issues. Others still can lead to a degradation of the body's ability to function effectively. Overall, the type of the chronic illness can range greatly. In fact, all of the conditions that you will be reading about within this book can be considered chronic.

Nevertheless, let's take a brief look over three common chronic illnesses that people suffer from. As you go through these illnesses, try to identify the ways that they may be related to the vagus nerve.

Though it is not commonly considered a disease, obesity is more than a superficial occurrence—it is not just about looks, but about health as well. When you are obese, you risk developing a myriad of other health issues, ranging from heart disease to cancer. Those who suffer from obesity have excess body fat, and for some people, that weight is harder to shed than for others.

Obesity has all sorts of risk factors—it could be caused due to hormones, genetics, or simply bad habits, such as eating too much without exercising. Oftentimes, those who are obese eat more than those who are of healthy sizes, and may also eat due to their own feelings as a way to sort of self-soothe.

Diabetes itself refers to several disease that all alter how your body processes glucose—the primary substance used for energy by your body. Typically, when considering diabetes, you will be looking at two disease: Type 1 diabetes and type 2 diabetes. These two diseases vary greatly. Women can also develop gestational diabetes as a result of a pregnancy.

These diseases can wreak havoc on the human body, directly influencing how the body functions, heals, and regulates itself. Considering that we primarily eat to raise blood sugar in order to continue functioning at a normal level, having that disconnect and struggle for the body to regulate accordingly can lead to massive issues. The body sometimes struggles to function and heal, and if left untreated without care taken to treat the diseases, it can lead to neuropathy and eventually death. Blood sugar levels that rise too much can cause comas and even death.

The vagus nerve relates to all three of these illnesses—if you stop and look at some of the symptoms, you can start to piece this together on your own. Alzheimer's disease sufferers start to see legitimate progress with their cognitive abilities and anxiety related symptoms when they have their vagal nerve stimulated. While it is not entirely known why, it is known that several of the precursor risk factors to Alzheimer's are related to the vagus nerve—high blood pressure can make it more likely that it is developed later in life, which as you know, is linked to the vagus nerve.

When it comes to obesity, the vagus nerve regulates the digestive system. This means that the individual's digestive system is going to respond to the vagus nerve. It will entirely regulate based on feedback by the vagus nerve—the nerve will determine whether your brain receives the message that you have eaten your fill or not, which then impacts how much you eat. Obesity, ultimately, is usually associated with the vagus nerve losing sensitivity for some reason—having a poorly responding vagus nerve means that the signal that tells your brain that you are full is too quiet. Effectively, then, the vagus nerve's dysfunction can, in some instances, be attributed to the obesity.

Diabetes, then, can also be closely linked to the vagus nerve—if it regulates the diet, and some diabetes can be induced via diet, it stands to reason that diabetes is sometimes caused by the vagus nerve. Beyond just that, however, the vagus nerve, at least in mice, has been found to provide information to the brain about the glucose levels within the body. Therefore, if that informational circuit were to get damaged, it would become vastly more difficult to regulate whether the individual had a sufficient level of glucose in the blood.

Vagus Nerve and Inflammation

As simply put as possible, inflammation is swelling in the body. The area swells and warms and the body then knows to focus on healing that particular area. It could be some sort of injury or an infection from bacteria— no matter what it is, inflammation is how the body triggers itself to go and pay attention to the area in order to ensure it heals.

Without this inflammation, the body would not heal in a timely manner—your broken bone would never mend itself and your infections would be free to run rampant like an invasive species, destroying the area around them and quickly spreading to infect more of you.

Effectively, if your body is a vehicle for your mind, think of your inflammation as your maintenance system. It will go through, flag areas of concern, and then work on healing it. Of course, it can also be overzealous as well. As with all things in life, there is such thing as too much of a good thing—when left to its own devises and free to worsen as much as it wants, inflammation can cause massive issues. It can lead to all sorts of autoimmune diseases and disorders, in which the body begins to attack itself instead of only on harmful injuries and foreign bodies.

Effectively, as you can see dictated in the previously provided table with a step-by-step play of the inflammation cycle, it is meant to directly protect and heal the body from any infections. In fighting off the bacteria and viruses that are causing problems, the body is providing itself with a chance to repair damage before it festers and gets out of hand. This means that the individual is able to recover from infections that, if left ignored and untreated, could be fatal.

This proper response leads to people with entirely normal, functioning inflammation levels when it is necessary. For example, when you are injured or you get a minor infection, that inflammation is necessary. The body regulates itself. However, for some people, this inflammation response can be largely suppressed, leading to immunodeficiency. Those whose response is too strong, on the other hand, can find themselves struggling with highly responsive inflammatory responses that attack themselves.

Vagus Nerve and PTSD

People can suffer from PTSD after a car accident, losing someone close to them unexpectedly, losing a home, particularly when unexpected and violent, being the victim of some sort of assault, physical or sexual, enduring abuse, or really anything else that would potentially be traumatic for the individual.

Those who struggle with PTSD often find themselves facing flashbacks and recurring intrusive thoughts that can make coping effectively nearly impossible. They essentially get stuck in a cycle in which the brain cannot properly process and handle the traumas, and as a result, they find that they are unable to finally get themselves out of fight-flight-freeze mode and back into rest-and-digest mode. Because of this, those suffering from PTSD can seem especially volatile, especially in situations or contexts that are even vaguely reminiscent of the trauma they endured. In fact, even something as simple as a scent, a word, or the way something is said can trigger an attack if the individual is reminded of the trauma in some way.

These suicidal thoughts, tendencies, and ideations should be taken incredibly seriously and as a medical emergency. If you feel like you are having suicidal thoughts or feelings, it is important that you reach out to someone you can trust—perhaps a friend, family member, or spouse, and ask for help. You do not have to feel this way forever, and there is no reason to create a permanent solution to something that is temporary at worst. If you have no one you can reach out to, please do not hesitate to call your emergency services for help.

Keep in mind just how intricately linked to fight-flight-freeze and rest-and-digest the vagus nerve is and consider for a moment what PTSD is. It involves regulating the fear response, as well as telling the body when that fear response is appropriate. If PTSD is largely due to an inability to regulate those responses to the trauma, it stands to reason that the two are intricately linked to each other.

Evidence has shown that those suffering from PTSD do, in fact, show a diminished functioning of the parasympathetic nervous system, implying that it is not regulating itself effectively and because the body is never able to put the individual into rest-and-digest mode due to the lack of the parasympathetic activity triggering the proper hormones, instead the individual is stuck in fight-flight-freeze mode. Consider the symptoms for a moment: Feeling guarded and afraid are two major symptoms of PTSD, and both of them are directly related to the sympathetic nervous system being in control. Now consider insomnia, which is an inability to sleep. That inability to sleep is related to the fact that the body cannot get itself out of fight-flight-freeze mode. During that time, the individual is stuck awake, no matter how tired he or she may be feeling, all because the body is unable to relax enough to effectively sleep.

When the parasympathetic nervous system takes control defensively, as is common in PTSD, the body shuts down on itself. It overcorrects, leading to a numbness or freeze response. Then, with people with PTSD, they are reacting with an overactive or underactive vagus nerve, leading to that feeling of shutting down and being numb or unable to feel joy.

Vagus Nerve and Sleep Disorders

Despite common perceptions, sleep is not just a time for the brain to turn off for the night—it actually facilitates several different processes that are necessary for proper functioning. Sleep is largely found to have three key functions: It allows the body to recover, it facilitates the memory consolidation process, and is related to the immune system. Each of these three functions are crucial, and are so important that the human body happens to spend about 1/3 of each and every day actively asleep, not counting the time preparing to sleep and getting comfortable in order to all asleep. Sleep is important, and if you do not give it to yourself, your body will eventually force the point— you will fall asleep at some point, even if you try to stay awake in the first place.

When you sleep, your body repairs itself. Your cells are literally attempting to regenerate themselves, and the rest of your body slows down so energy can be redirected to those cells that need it, allowing them to heal themselves. As you sleep as well, your mind begins to consolidate all of the memories you have made throughout the day, also allowing you to effectively learn better. It has been found that those who sleep shortly after being taught to play a video game tend to do better than those who stay up late in an attempt to practice longer to develop skills quicker. Lastly, when you sleep while sick, your body is able to better produce cytokines, allowing the body to then fight off the infection quicker, which is quite likely why people get so tired when they are sick.

Sleep disorders, then, are the creation of some change in the way that you are sleeping, and these changes are typically quite negative. They can involve sleeping too much, not enough, or simply not getting restful sleep in the first place. The end result to not getting enough sleep, however, is the creation of all sorts of health issues. Sleep deprivation itself can quite literally be dangerous, especially because the signs of sleep deprivation can be so extreme.

Some of these symptoms include mood irregularities, creating irritation and depression. They can lead to cognitive impairments, causing a struggle to concentrate on any tasks at hand and forgetfulness, as well as a struggle to learn anything new, and more.

Vagus nerve stimulation has been used to treat epilepsy, in which an implant electrically stimulates the vagus nerve. However, it has also been found to have a direct impact on the ability to regulate and has been linked to increased daytime alertness, meaning that the individual, especially if they are suffering from narcolepsy or something similar, will be able to stay awake longer.

The problem, however, is that it has been found that the vagus nerve stimulator, in particular the electrical stimulator, can cause an increase in apnea. This apnea can also worsen the occurrence rate of seizures in general, making it difficult to determine whether stimulating the vagus nerve electrically is a good fit for those struggling with sleep apnea or other sleep disorders.

Vagus Nerve and Gerd

Hydrochloric acid is one of the most important areas of optimal digestion in the abdomen. Acid does of course have a variety of functions, if they are incompletely done, then acid reflux, stomach pain and indigestion are temporarily present.

In the long term, he or she may have IBS, food allergies, food intolerance, mineral and vitamin deficiency and certain autoimmune diseases.

The main characteristics of acid are the identification of proteins, minerals and vitamins. The acid also kills parasites and bacteria in order to prevent them from reaching the bloodstream and intestines.

With far too little acidity, the food can stay longer in the stomach until it can even absorb and process the food (the belly is a muscle) while it is hard for the stomach to cause a little fluid up the esophagus.

That's what many people see as cardiac (also called GERD). If the acidity level was certainly higher the valve would not have closed between the esophagus and the stomach.

The food stays in a tummy with low acidity for a long time, and the person suffers from bloating.

If the half-digested food continues to the small intestine, further food breakdown is complicated, because the gut cannot process it in its form. This is when abdominal pain happens.

In addition, the meals contain microscopic, undigested components that fill the intestine and bloodstream structure. Headache and food intolerance and allergy may result. This condition is known as leaking intestines.

If you possibly experience these symptoms and they are triggered by too low acidity, taking drugs to further reduce acidity can exacerbate the problem.

If you have too little or too much acidity, fire one or two cubes between meals of apple cider vinegar. You can often get it straight or mix it in a bottle with a small quantity of h2o. If this prevents heartburn, the lack of acid production is your concern.

It is estimated that about 90% of people with similar conditions and cardiovascular disease have far too low acidity.

The main reason why the abdomen does not produce enough acid is simply that messages from mind to abdomen are blocked. The brain sends signals throughout the vagus nerve on the stomach (and other organs).

This specific nerve starts in the brain and passes the entire process to the intestines on the chest. With some people this particular nerve has been punched into the neck during birth, which also prevents an element of acid production communication on the stomach.A kinesiologist or chiropractor with a noninvasive small procedure which takes a few minutes can easily freely release the vagus nerve. It's worth taking the time to do this; your entire digestion will boost considerably. However, if you're a smoker the smoking addiction will be gone and several allergies may decrease as electrical resistance.

Vagus Nerve and Hunger

Hunger is only one major cause of the vagus nerve. But if you immerse yourself in PubMed, you will find that vagus nerve dysfunction is related to many other issues.

That's because the vagus nerve often helps you to control inflammation and almost all chronic conditions include inflammation. Are subtly relaxing nerve signals anti-inflammatory in the brain? It indicates that the brain activates the stress reaction and reduces the production of inflammatory cytokines.

The results are a little difficult to unwrap, as the vagus nerve is two-way, and there are plenty of complicated feedback loops between the gut and the brain (remember that the vagus nerve works both ways!).

But for the people who are simply worried about enhancing their health, the actual mechanism may be less precious than the end result: the vagus nerve effect of inflammation has a cardiovascular health impact and then vagus nerve stimulation may minimize cardiovascular events.

This particular study is extremely interesting: the treatment of vagal nerve stimulation-prone rats with diabetes reduces anxiety and sensitivity to insulin. This is an overwhelming proportion of evidence that diabetes and depression can both start in the gut.

If a bad food program affects the vagus nerve resistance, it could also affect each of these diseases. This can be one reason why wellness is such an enormous health game.

But if a lazy food plan will decrease the vagus nerve's resistance, perhaps a great diet plan will help to heal. While not using a junk food diet, a little more basic work is available here. There are obviously not many diets and vagus nerve reports. Although it is something to start with and it can support the key ways the gut, the human brain and the rest of your body tend to be linked.

Chapter 5: Substances and other things That May Interfere with the Vagus Nerve functionality

It is good to know about the many foods that help you improve the vagus nerve. It helps you manage your diet and change your eating habits.

But that is just one part of the equation. There is the part where we are thinking about adding more of something and then there is the part where we have to reduce some of the good stuff. Think about it. It does not matter how many salads and greens we eat if we only end up heading over to KFC and ordering a nice 10-piece chicken bucket.

The same principle applies to the vagus nerve as well. We need to watch what we eat, both by including healthy food and removing harmful components.

Apart from the food we eat, we also need to watch out for other substances that enter our bodies. While you might think that these substances do not have any effect on the vagus nerve, you might be surprised by the results. Let us look at some of these substances.

Botox

Breathing is essential for life. We take in oxygen that fills up our lungs and gets carried into our blood. We exhale carbon dioxide, by-products of a successful breathing process.

But what exactly tells our body to breathe? Is it our mind? Our brain?

Well, our brain is definitely involved, but there is much more to breathing than that. You see, what tells our lungs to not stop breathing and suffocate us is a certain neurotransmitter called acetylcholine. Guess what part of the body is responsible for the creation of these neurotransmitters?

What does botox have to do with any of this? Isn't that a cosmetic substance? It's applied to the skin and not into the lungs, so there does not seem to be any connection.

The truth is not in the process, but the chemicals released by the process. You see, when you use botox, you inject the stuff into your muscles. This ends up interrupting the production of acetylcholine in your body. Which is why botox can be potentially dangerous to you.

Too much botox can eventually lead to a deficit of acetylcholine in your body and at the same time, a blockage of the vagus nerve. The only conclusion to all of this is the end of our lives.

While that might sound grim, it is a reminder of how to maintain control over what you do. It helps you to understand that some things should not be taken in excess.

Certain Antibiotics

Now I am not telling you to completely stop taking antibiotics. When you have a certain strain of bacteria affecting your body and causing all sorts of damage, then you need antibiotics to deal with the situation. In short, listen to your doctor.

But at the same time, the name says it all. Antibiotics attack the bacteria in our body. The way they do this means they don't focus on getting rid of just a particular bacteria, but related bacteria as well. This is why they could cause harm to some of the useful bacteria that live in our body.

That still does not mean that you have to skip out on the antibiotics. So what else can someone do? Is there an alternative?

This is where probiotics come into play. The main purpose of probiotics is to add useful bacteria into the body. This becomes useful when you are consuming antibiotics. For example, let's say that a particular antibiotic has removed a certain bacteria from the body. Using a probiotic replenishes that particular bacteria.

Doctors are careful about this and usually prescribe probiotics to their patients if the need arises. However, remember that if probiotics are not needed, then you don't have to ask for one. Your doctor is usually aware of the risks of prescribing certain antibiotics and if he or she feels that you might need to take something else along with your medications, then that is usually given to you. If you feel doubtful, always ask your doctor for more clarification. They would be happy to explain to you.

Heavy Metals

When you get a high dose of a certain heavy metal, then you might suffer the symptoms below:

- It might disrupt your brain functions and you might end up feeling lost or confused.
- Numbness in certain parts of the body
- Nausea and vomiting
- In certain instances, you might pass out completely.

How does mercury harm the vagus nerve? Well, let's just say that you could consider botox and mercury as partners in crime because they both operate the same way; they affect the production of acetylcholine in the body. This in turn prevents the body from sending proper signals to the lungs to breathe. Is there a way to prevent mercury poisoning? Of course there is.

Keep in mind that trace amounts of it might be found in numerous food that we eat and that low levels are usually ignored or managed without difficulty by the body. But some of the foods that you can avoid in order to prevent a higher level of mercury in your body are:

- Fish that has high levels of mercury
- Any additional supplements or dietary pills with high mercury

Excessive Sugar

Excess sugar is bad for a lot of reasons. Apart from the fact that it is one of the biggest causes of diabetes, it is also harmful because it causes chronic inflammation. Such inflammation creates disruptions on the body's cellular feedback loops and other signaling pathways. What this means is that different parts of the body are not able to communicate with each other well. Of course, communication is the primary function of the nervous system.

It is also for this reason that when high amounts of sugar cause blurry vision, difficulty thinking, and fatigue, the body thinks that you are getting a panic attack and falsely activates the fight-or-flight process. But the reality is that you are not having a panic attack. Your body does not realize this because it is taking time for one part of the body to tell the other that it's just a false alarm.

In order to prevent such disruptions in communication, make sure you reduce the intake of sugar. If you are someone who cannot keep away from that delicious Hershey's bar of chocolate, then either choose to have it in moderation or, in the case of diabetes or any indicators of diabetes, you have no other choice but to skip it entirely.

Chapter 6: How to activate and stimulate your Vagus Nerve

For some people, they may find that their dysfunction requires electrical stimulation.

This is where the ever so handy vagus nerve stimulator device comes in. As mentioned, this device is similar to that of a pacemaker for heart patients. This is often one of the first recommended treatments for a vagus nerve with severe damage along the way. You can also try one of the main at home methods that have been previously mentioned during the book and within our passive activities list.

You can treat vagus nerve damage at home with care on the basis that it has not reached a life threatening severity. Choosing exactly which method works for your body to maintain your health and a healthy lifestyle is incredibly important in the long run as this is your body that you need to take care of. Gentle exercise can be incredibly good for you and will not harm you in any way as long as it is done properly, especially while your vagus nerve is healing from some sort of trauma. If you give any of our more advanced, yoga-type exercises a try and you are a beginner, try to find a teacher-led class that may be able to give you a hand when you are upside down and looking something like a pretzel. If you are battling with any of these exercises, then a teacher will be able to guide and help you and correct any poses so that you may reap all the benefits in the long run from the exercise. Choosing the correct form of treatment is also something that should be discussed in detail with your medical practitioner.

It would also be a good idea to get somebody trusted, such as a close friend or family member, who could also help you through the challenging times ahead and keep you on track.

Sometimes it's almost easy to say that we can combat this by simply keeping control of our vagus nerve and strengthening it through stimulation or even by seeing a doctor, but a big part of the healing process is also to have a good support system at your back. When you have people who are aware of the problem and are able to give you emotional support along the way, you will be far more likely to stay calm during the process and know that you aren't alone, which will also keep you on the right track when completely giving up starts to look good. Find an emotional partner who can hold you accountable and tackle this problem head-on.

Understanding that you can use your vagus nerve for self-regulation, then, you are able to develop the capacity to activate your vagus nerve at will. You will be able to encourage your body to trigger that parasympathetic reaction at will. Your body will naturally calm. Your heart rate and blood pressure will regulate. Your body will begin to rest. This will lead to more restful sleep, allowing you to better digest the food that you do ingest.

Regular stimulation of your vagus nerve will keep it working well and will improve vagal tone. Like muscles, the nerve requires regular exercise to keep it toned and to function at its best. While diet and being grateful can help your vagal tone, there are quite a few other ways to stimulate the nerve.

Even when your vagus nerve is inhibited by sympathetic responses, they are methods you can use to stimulate and restore parasympathetic responses in your body. Some of these methods include:

Healthy Diet

The Vagus nerve is surrounded by a protective sheath of myelin that protects the vagus nerve from injury and ensures that nerve impulses are transmitted properly. Good myelin health is, therefore, important for the proper function of your Vagus nerve.

The health of the myelin sheath, however, starts to deteriorate as we age, meaning that the vagus nerve becomes more susceptible to injury and malfunction the older we get. This protective layer, myelin, is a lipid-based compound, and we can help mitigate the effects of aging on the myelin by observing a healthy diet which should be characterized by:

Fruits such as strawberries, kiwis, blackcurrants, oranges, guavas, papayas, and lemons are great sources of vitamin C that you can incorporate into your diet. Vegetables such as broccoli, brussels sprouts, bell peppers, and kale are also rich in vitamin- C.

You can improve many aspects of your health simply by eating correctly, but did you know that this also has a massive effect on your vagus nerve? I didn't realize until after I had already changed my eating habits that there were some other benefits to this lifestyle, including boosting vagal tone.

It turns out that what you eat and the bacteria in your digestive tract actually affect how your brain functions. The bacteria in your gut can get upset or become imbalanced when you take antibiotics or other types of medicines. That's exactly what happened to me. So when my friend told me to take probiotics, she was actually on the right track. It just takes more than a few bottles of kombucha to fix the gut.

What Foods Should You Eat?

The types of foods you eat are very important, but some are more so. Here are some foods that should be included in your daily diet:

- Fermented Food: Fermented foods include healthy microbes and bacteria, so they can help restore your digestive tract bacteria if it has been depleted. Things like sauerkraut, cheese, kefir, kombucha, and yogurt are some of the more common fermented foods. However, you can also make fermented salsa, ketchup, and many other delicious, gut-boosting foods at home.

- Foods High in Fiber: You want to keep things moving and one of the signs that your gut is not healthy is constipation. It makes sense then to eat fiber, but there's another good reason for this . . . prebiotics. Your high fiber foods contain prebiotics that will help good gut bacteria flourish and reduce your stress levels. High fiber foods include anything made with whole grains, seeds, fruits and vegetables, and nuts.
- Calcium: Known as the bone-building mineral, calcium helps protect the body against diseases like diabetes and cancer. It's also an essential part of keeping your nervous system and cardiovascular system functioning properly, which includes your vagus nerve. Calcium is one of the nutrients that the body cannot produce, so you need to eat it. You'll find calcium in dairy products, dark green

leafy vegetables like kale or broccoli, and in canned fish with softened bones.

- **Magnesium:** Without magnesium, the heart cannot function as well as it should. In fact, this mineral is an essential part of regulating the circulatory system. It helps the heart contract correctly, manages heart rhythm and prevents many cardiac issues. It can be found in nuts and seeds, green leafy vegetables like kale and spinach, figs, avocado, bananas, and seafood in general. Legumes such as beans and peas are also rich in magnesium.
- **Sodium:** Chances are you've heard that salt is bad for you all your life. It's a common misconception and, while too much sodium isn't great for the body, it is necessary for your body to function. Whole grain bread, cured meats, and chicken are all excellent sources of sodium. You can also use sea salt or Himalayan salt in your food.

- Potassium: Potassium is found in every tissue throughout the body and is responsible for a number of functions. It helps keep the bowels moving and helps muscles contract. Potassium is also essential for nerve transmission . . . which makes it very useful for keeping the vagus nerve functioning correctly. This mineral can be found in citrus fruits, dates, spinach, beans and cantaloupe, among other foods.
- Phosphorus: Calcium and phosphorus work together to create strong, healthy bones and teeth. Phosphorus is also useful in managing energy and keeping your vagus nerve healthy. It's also important in regulating hormones. Any excess phosphorus is eliminated by the kidneys, as long as they are healthy. It's found in chicken, eggs, cheese, canned sardines, milk, and sunflower seeds, among other things.
- Omega-3s: Omega-3 fats are essential for brain health and can also help your

digestive system out. You'll find them in oily fish like salmon, flaxseeds, canola oil, soy oil, and nuts and seeds. Not only will these fats help your brain and gut, but they're also very useful in boosting energy, improving the immune system, and increasing the efficiency of your hormone-producing glands.

- **Polyphenol:** Polyphenols are chemicals produced by plants and processed by the bacteria in your digestive tract. They increase the number of healthy bacteria and have been linked to the elimination of brain fog. You can find polyphenols in green tea, coffee, olive oil, and cocoa, as well as cloves, beans, nuts, soy, and berries, among other foods.

- **Tryptophan:** You probably know of tryptophan as the amino acid that is found in turkey, but it is also readily available in eggs and cheese. This amino acid does more than make you sleepy on Thanksgiving. It actually converts to serotonin, which is the neurotransmitter responsible for making you feel happy.

Each of these nutrients is important, so make sure you include them in your diet. There is something to be said for eating a varied diet, though, so don't obsess too much about it. Include plenty of the vegetables and foods mentioned above and you should get everything you need in your diet.

You can eat plenty of great food, but there are a few foods that should be avoided, as well. Make sure you know what these are so you can plan your food around them.

Foods to avoid include those that promote inflammation. Refined carbs, like white bread, tend to inflame the body, as do fried foods and sodas. In fact, anything with refined sugar can cause serious health issues and the additional inflammation boosts immune response and lowers vagal tone. If you're not sure if a food is good for you or not, look at the ingredient list. If there are more ingredients than just the basic foods, you should probably skip it. For example, apple puree that includes a long list of chemicals isn't the best choice and won't provide as much nutrition as puree made with actual apples and nothing else.

Meal planning can help you ensure that your meals are full of beneficial foods. When you make last-minute meals, you're more likely to grab whatever is quick and easy. You are also less likely to have what you need on hand for a healthy meal. Instead, write up a menu for the week and then shop according to that menu. It's a good idea to plan for at least a few super simple meals. This lessens the likelihood that you'll skip or order takeout.

Another way to help ensure that you eat well is to make food ahead. It's simple to eat healthily when you always have a big bowl of salad in the fridge. You will also find that you can easily put together a great meal if you keep some basics cooked and on hand, such as beans, prepared chicken or beef, brown rice, etc. Make sure you also have healthy snacks readily available to grab when you're hungry. The easier you make it to eat well, the less likely you are to grab fast food or something that is too processed to be good for you.

In the end, a balanced diet is the best thing for you, but as long as you focus on eating foods that will boost gut health and avoiding foods that increase inflammation. Your gut health will have a major impact on your nervous system.

Expose yourself to cold/Cold therapy

To use cold therapy to activate your vagus nerve, there are various techniques you can use. For example, you can simply turn the water to cold for the last two minutes of your regular shower. Alternatively, splashing ice-cold water on your face will also have a positive effect on your vagus nerve. Taking a walk outside when the temperature is low can also help you activate the vagus nerve.

If you feel that your body is up for the challenge, you can also try taking ice baths. This will involve putting three bags of ice into a half-filled tub and getting in once the ice is melted. To do this safely, ensure that you do not stay in the ice bath for an extended period of time. Taking a hot beverage after the ice bath will be effective in warming you up again.

Cold temperatures have been found to have an effect on reducing stress, anxiety, and stimulating the gastric nerves through vagal stimulation. When you feel yourself getting anxious, losing concentration, or simply getting worn out mentally, splash some cold water on your face or just take a break and walk outside in the cold for a while; it may not solve your problem, but it will definitely calm you down and clear your mind.

As you cool yourself off, exposing yourself to sudden acute cold, you are able to cause several different effects—you are able to speed up the metabolism while also causing any swelling, inflammation, or other discomfort to lessen. This is exactly why you are told to put ice on a swollen or otherwise inflamed part of your body—the ice alleviates the swelling. The exposure to the cold can also increase the rest that you get, allowing your sleep to improve in quality, which is why many people in northern countries have a tendency to leave their children sleeping on a cold winter day.

When you want to do this for yourself, you effectively trigger your body to constrict the blood vessels, just like you did in the Valsalva maneuver, which then enables the body to start regulating itself. Beyond the myriad of other benefits, you will trigger your heart rate to slow down through exposing yourself to the cold for a short period of time.

Nevertheless, short, acute exposures to this sort of sudden drop of temperature can do wonders to regulate your vagus nerve's activation. Of course, there are several different ways that you can activate your vagus nerve through exposure to the cold.

One such way is through ice baths—this is often seen by athletes, especially after a long workout session. In this, you are doing exactly what it sounds like—you are bathing in ice water. You may do this in an icy cold swimming pool or bathtub, for example, or you may even go through the process of dipping yourself into an icy cold river or lake on a winter day. No matter how you go through this process, remember that you are doing so for a brief period—you do not want to inflict harm, but rather go through the cold long enough to reap the benefits.

When you do this, you will see several benefits—you will find yourself feeling far more awake, thanks to the sudden shock to your system. This will also make you take deeper breaths, which activates your vagus nerve as already discussed. As you do this as well, you will see that you willpower increases—while this may not necessarily be directly related to any of the illnesses that have been discussed thus far, it is still a pretty cool benefit! You may even see weight loss as your body makes it a point to create brown fat instead of the usual fat that is developed. Brown fat is the fat that infants have naturally—it is a massive user of energy, which allows for the extra burning of calories.

Another method that has grown popular lately that may be a bit less accessible to you but is still legitimate nevertheless is through cryo therapy. This involves you standing in a small, enclosed space and being blasted with cold air. Think of this as an air conditioner in a small space on steroids—it is meant to be extreme cold for a short period of time. This may not help you if you are not in an area where this is an option, or if you are unwilling or unable to spend the money that such a therapy would cost, but it has still become popular.

The most accessible of the options, especially year-round, is through using cold water that you splash on your face when you feel like you need to calm down or self-regulate. If you feel overly emotional, as if you are panicking or anxious, or generally just out of sorts, try splashing cold water on your face or taking a quick cold shower. Doing so triggers the same effect as the previous methods, but it is free and easily accessible, no matter where you are. You can even go through this process out and about, simply by entering a restroom and using their sink for a moment to cool yourself off before continuing on with your day.

Intermittent fasting

Intermittent fasting refers to a nutrition plan where you eat for a certain period of time, followed by a period of abstaining from food, which is the fasting phase. Intermittent fasting means fasting in intervals. For example, you can fast for 18 hours in a day and restrict your feeding period to 6 hours.

When you fast, the vagus nerve detects the inevitable drop that occurs in glucose levels when we go without eating. Once it has detected the drop in blood glucose, the vagus nerve signals the brain to reduce metabolism, which has the effect of slowing down the heart rate and switching of the body's sympathetic responses of fight or flight. In this way, fasting is effective in stimulating vagal activity.

Intermittent fasting has become one of the more popular weight loss methods because it is effective in insulin regulation, and therefore, promotes fat burning in the body. This method, apart from the obvious benefits in terms of weight management, is an effective way to activate the vagus nerve.

To benefit from the effects of fasting in stimulating your vagus nerve, you can opt for moderate fasting plans of 16 hours or 18 hours a couple of times in a week. The ultimate effect is that fasting by stimulating your vagus nerve will also have positive effects on your mental clarity and overall ability to manage anxiety and stress.

Physical Exercise

Getting sufficient exercise is incredibly important for everyone's overall health and wellbeing, but what sort of effect does it have on the vagus nerve itself? Exercise increases growth hormone within your brain as well as reversing cognitive decline in the human brain function.

This helps to stimulate the vagus nerve which in turn will also benefit your gut flow, heart rate, and muscles that get stimulated as you exercise.

There is no getting away from the fact that physical exercise has multiple beneficial effects on our physical health. It not only improves cardiovascular health; it also helps in fat burning and weight management. Exercise has also been proven to be effective in combating stress and anxiety. When we engage in physical exercise, the body release chemicals called endorphins that have an uplifting effect on the mood and are responsible for the feel-good after effect of exercising.

If that's not enough to get you up and moving, physical exercise is an effective way to stimulate your vagus nerve and enhance your vagal tone. Exercise stimulates your vagus nerve resulting in enhanced mental clarity and stimulation of the brain's growth hormone.

When it comes to stimulating the vagus nerve using physical exercise, there is no limit to the type of exercises you can use. Lifting weights, jogging, taking brisk walks, aerobics, and even yoga will all help in boosting vagal activity and promoting the body's self-healing mechanisms.

Any kind of exercise can be beneficial, so pick something you enjoy. If you like the exercise you're doing, you will be more likely to keep it up. A few activities you might like to try include:

- Walking: Just a stroll around the park or the block can help boost your activity level.
- Swimming: This is a good low-impact exercise for those with limited mobility and it builds muscle tone, too.
- Cycling: Jump on a bike and start pedaling to boost lung capacity, lose weight, and tone your nervous system.
- Hiking: This is a good option for getting into your social connections, too, since hiking is best done with a friend or two.
- Running/jogging: You don't have to run a race (though that's fun, too), but getting out and moving fast will give you a vagal tone boost.
- Weight lifting: If going places isn't something you enjoy, try weight lifting to tone both muscles and the vagus nerve.
- Yoga: Build tone with stretches and add in some social elements, too, if you take a class.

- Aerobics: Another great way to get moving is with an aerobics class, or you can do a video class at home.
- Dancing: Who doesn't love dancing? Hit the clubs or just stay home and dance your way around the house. It all counts.
- Kayaking: Get out on the water and get some exercise for a relaxing vagal tone increase.
- Martial arts: You can learn to defend yourself and boost your vagal tone at the same time.
- Gymnastics: You will learn to stretch and move, so it's a two for one kind of deal.
- Sports: If you enjoy playing basketball, soccer, or something else, you'll find that playing a sport on a team gives you a real energy boost.

There's no limit to the types of movement you can try. If something doesn't work for you, move on to something else.

If you find that exercise is tough for you to keep up with, even when it's something you enjoy, there are a few ways to ensure you keep it up. There's nothing wrong with a little added motivation to keep you moving.

- Find an accountability partner. Working out with someone else, even if it's just a walking partner, is particularly helpful. If you make a date to meet with someone to exercise, you'll be more likely to keep the date, rather than bailing at the last minute. Alternatively, you can just have someone that you report to each day, even if they're long-distance. Having to check-in will give you more reason to do what you said you would.
- Sign up for classes. If you spend money on classes, you'll likely keep up with them. After all, you wouldn't want to throw away the money. Just make sure it's something you actually want to do. It makes little sense to take a karate class if you hate martial arts, for example. There are so many different physical classes available that there's no shortage of things to learn.

- Join a team. Really need some motivation? Consider joining a sports team. Whether you want to play baseball locally or jump into dragon boating, a team will keep you going when you don't feel like moving, simply because there are other people depending on you. For those who are competitive, a team sport can be very enjoyable and may get you moving even more than usual.
- Hire a trainer. A personal trainer is an extra expense, but if you can afford it, you'll have someone to push you to your limit. I found that a personal trainer really helped me get past the exercise hump. When I couldn't push myself, it helped to have someone else there to push me.
- Get a dog. Not only does a dog make a great companion and give unconditional love, but it will also need to be walked. You can't get away with skipping the walks or you'll have a mess in your house.

The extra motivation to go out might be just what you need to get moving.

It can also help to reward yourself once you reach a certain goal, such as running a distance in a certain amount of time or lifting a certain amount of weight. You choose your reward, but it should be something that will motivate you.

Massage

Massages can be so relaxing and effective in relieving tension and stress in the body. It is, therefore, no surprise that they can be used as a means of activating the vagus nerve. One of the most effective massages when it comes to vagal activation is reflexology massages.

A reflexology massage involves the application of different amounts of pressure to different parts of the body, specifically, the feet, hands, and ears. A reflexology massage will increase the activity of the vagus nerve, inhibit sympathetic fight or flight responses and even slow down the heart rate. This means that this type of massages soothes the body into a relaxed state that promotes vagal function and mental clarity.

Massaging the neck area is also effective in stimulating the vagus nerve by applying pressure on the carotid sinus. Pressure massages are also effective in vagal stimulation. When you are feeling tense or having a bad day, visiting a good massage therapist will help you to relax and reduce your anxiety and stress levels. Certain types of massage can stimulate the vagus nerve. Reflexology has been shown to stimulate the vagus nerve and improve both vagal tone and reduce anxiety. Foot massages can lower the fight or flight response and engage the vagus nerve, but other types of massages are also beneficial. This is a very physical method of stimulating the vagus nerve and it can be terrifically effective if you use it right. Besides, who doesn't enjoy a good massage?

Your massage can be in just one area of your body or you can go for a full body massage. Have a loved one do it for you or get a professional to stimulate that nerve. Whatever you choose, make sure it's relaxing and enjoyable. If you hate having your feet touched, for example, you're not going to get as much benefit from a foot massage as you would if you enjoyed it.

Face massages that include the neck are excellent for stimulating the vagus nerve, but even a good shoulder massage from a friend can give you the benefits you're looking for. If you need an excuse to have more massages, now you have it. It's all for your vagal tone.

Sleep hygiene

Getting enough sleep is important for good physical and mental health. When we haven't slept well during the night, our ability to function well the next day is impaired because we are not rested, and the lack of rest results in a kind of mental fogginess that hinders clarity of thought. Sleeping also allows the body to activate its self-healing mechanisms and rejuvenate itself by renewing worn-out cells and tissues.

When your sleep quality is bad, then your immunity, mental, and emotional health are likely to suffer. The relationship between sleep and vagal tone is cyclic. This means that getting sufficient sleep will boost your vagal tone. On the other hand, when your vagus nerve is not functioning properly, you are likely to experience poor quality of sleep and may even end up suffering from insomnia.

Probiotics

The communication between the gut and the brain is facilitated by the vagus nerve through the gut-brain axis. This axis basically links emotional and cognitive brain centers to the gut functions. Our gut plays host to a variety of microbes that are important in enabling the breakdown of compounds during the digestion process. These microbes communicate to the brain using the vagus nerve, and hence the presence of "good bacteria" in our gut is one way of enhancing brain activity.

While the thought of ingesting bacteria may sound revolting, it is important to note that not all microorganisms cause diseases. In fact, most are quite harmless and are actually useful in digestive processes in the gut. Microbes are a natural part of the ecosystem in our gut and actually play a role in improving digestion, preventing infection by hindering the development of disease-causing microorganisms, and boosting the immune system.

The good news is that probiotic-rich foods are easily available and should be pretty easy to incorporate into your diet.

They include:

- Yogurt – this healthy drink is made by the fermentation of milk by gut-friendly bacteria. There are natural and sugar-free varieties available for those watching their sugar intake.
- Sauerkraut – fermented cabbage has been a part of our diet for a long time because even in the olden days, its impact on gut health was well recognized. In addition to its probiotic content, sauerkraut is rich in vitamins such as Vitamins C and K and is rich in iron and manganese.
- Pickles-the fermentation of cucumbers to make pickles makes them a good source of probiotics and vitamins such as vitamin K.
- Cheese – cheese is a favorite addition to many dishes, and cheeses such as cottage cheese, mozzarella, and cheddar are all great sources of probiotics.

Yoga and Tai Chi

Studies have indicated that tai chi is effective in relieving chronic pain, improving overall body immunity, and promoting physical fitness. If you are seeking a means to activate your vagus nerve that comes with a host of other health benefits, then tai chi might be the way to go. Yoga, similarly to tai-chi, has beneficial effects when it comes to vagus nerve activation and in the reduction of stress and anxiety.

Practicing yoga encourages the mind and body to self soothe and get into a relaxed state, which is the ideal environment for the body's self-healing mechanism to work efficiently. Yoga typically incorporates physical exercise, meditation, and chanting to achieve mental and physical relaxation. There are different types of yoga that can be used to effectively activate the vagus nerve.

Good relationships

Good relationships are great for your immunity in terms of fighting off diseases and infections and are also vital for your psychological and emotional health.

Establishing great social networks and sound relationships with your family and friends will significantly decrease depressive tendencies and improve your overall ability to cope with stress, which, as we have seen is a big factor in physical and mental disorders.

We have a natural instinct for socialization that is part of the core of the human experience. We actively seek out relationships and connections with others to get a sense of belonging and oneness that is fostered by good relationships. Loneliness has, for a long time, been known to create a predisposition to depressive tendencies; this is because human contact is essential for our psychological wellbeing.

Your relationships have quite an effect on every aspect of your life, from health and mood to your self-confidence. It's best to surround yourself with positive relationships and people who lift you up. Doing this will not only make you feel happier, but it will also increase your vagus nerve tone and build your immune system.

The vagus nerve is connected to the nerves that hear and express speech. It is also responsible for oxytocin release, the hormone that is essential in human and animal bonding. It makes sense then that it can all affect you when speaking with someone else. If you are talking to someone who is negative or frightens you, then your stress response is activated, your heart rate goes up, and other unpleasant effects occur.

It has also been proven in studies that people who have a higher tone in their vagus nerve tend to be kinder and to bond better with others. If this isn't enough reason to be social, then you might want to look into making more human contact to find out what it feels like. However, this can also be activated when you are around animals. They love unconditionally and can make sure you get lots of positivity.

Regular interaction with other people can lift your spirits an amazing amount. It's easy these days to focus on just being online, but it doesn't count. The technology, while it allows us to communicate, doesn't allow for the person to person interaction that our brains and bodies require.

Getting a genuine hug from someone can tone your vagus nerve. If you get several hugs every day, you'll find that your mood improves. Both eye contact and human touch have massive effects on how toned your vagus nerve is. Every time you spend time with someone else, whether it's laughing over a cup of coffee or holding hands as you walk down the street, your vagus nerve is being stimulated.

Human connection can help you feel calmer, more positive, and improves your mood overall. The effects can last for days, in some situations.

Social engagement not only helps us relax, but it also effectively switches off our fight or flight responses by creating a safe and soothing environment for us to exist in. Maintaining good relationships will boost your vagal tone by stimulating your parasympathetic responses and by reducing stress, which tends to activate our fight or flight responses and inhibit vagal activity.

Meditation

Meditation is a mental exercise that exercises the mind through relaxation, heightened focus, and creating awareness. Meditation is similar to physical exercise, but for our minds rather than our bodies. Meditation enables us to exercise our minds and purify our thoughts.

Meditation is based on the following techniques:

- Concentration: This is achieved by focusing attention on a particular object that can be external or internal.
- Observation: This is where you concentrate on the sensations, feelings, and thoughts present in your body at that moment.
- Awareness: This is where you remain consciously aware of your own thoughts and feelings but without getting distracted or engaged physically or mentally.

In mindful meditation, the goal is typically to concentrate your mind on the thoughts, sensations, and emotions that you are experiencing in the present or current moment. It normally involves regulation of breathing, muscle and body relaxation, mental visualization, and a heightened awareness of the body and mind.

Did you know you can affect your health by just meditating? It's a known method of relaxing the body and mind, but if done regularly, you'll find it actually benefits your overall health. You'll find that anxiety is less likely to affect you and you won't immediately get anxious over small and unimportant things.

How you meditate depends on you, but many people enjoy listening to low music while they clear their mind and focus on their breathing. Emptying out your mind can be a clarifying experience and it has the added benefit of calming you and making you feel more centered as you go about your day.

If you find meditation confusing or difficult, consider using a guided meditation that you can listen to as you work on perfecting your technique. There are a number of free options on YouTube that can be used.

Meditation has the added benefit of using chanting or breathing techniques to help you relax, so you add another great method of activating your vagus nerve at the same time. You'll find that you have more energy and feel more balanced after a meditation session, too.

Mindfulness meditation is effective in stress reduction, cognitive therapy, as well as in the treatment of depression symptoms. The basic technique involved is easy to learn and can easily be done for about 10 minutes daily to obtain the benefits in terms of increasing your vagal tone.

Keep your stress levels in check

When it comes to activating your vagus nerve, stress will be your number one enemy. We have already established in previous chapters that for the parasympathetic systems to become activated, your body needs to be in a relaxed and rested state otherwise, your body's self-healing mechanism cannot be activated. Chronic stress keeps you in a constant state of fight or flight and inhibits the vagus nerve from functioning properly.

To avoid being constantly stressed, you can use any of the tools we have discussed, such as meditation, exercise, yoga, or even socially engagement. When you allow stress to dominate your life, the vagus nerve activity is overridden by the fight and flight responses that are activated when we are stressed. Managing stress can be an uphill task, but once you develop this skill, it will be one of the best things you can do for your body in terms of physical and mental wellbeing.

Disease Management

Chronic diseases such as rheumatoid arthritis, Alzheimer's, or epilepsy have no cure. However, stimulating the vagus nerve can help in making them more manageable and bearable for patients. The power of the vagus nerve in inhibiting chronic inflammation and turning down overactive immune responses means that it can greatly slow down degeneration in disorders such as arthritis and Alzheimer's.

In epilepsy, vagal stimulation therapy is now widely used in regulating the frequency, severity, and duration of seizures. This means that if you are suffering from any of these chronic illnesses, you can ask your doctor about including vagal stimulation therapy in your treatment plan to help alleviate some of the symptoms.

Weight Management

When your brain is not able to perceive fullness in the stomach, the natural consequence will be that you will tend to eat more. The communication between the gut and brain is facilitated by the vagus nerve, which means that if your vagus nerve is not functioning properly, your hunger and fullness cues will not be received correctly by the brain.

Activating the power of your vagus nerve can, therefore, help you in weight management by curbing overeating and facilitating proper digestive processing of food in the gut.

Gargling

Another fun way to stimulate the vagus nerve at home is to gargle with water. This action stimulates the muscles in the soft palate within your mouth which are directly being controlled by the vagus nerve.

You can even spice things up and hum while you are gargling to add to the effect that you will have on your vagus nerve to wake it up. Kids also find this particular kind of exercise most amusing and they can equally benefit from it being turned into a family game of sorts to see who can gargle the longest or loudest (letting them win will have an equally amusing effect).

Coffee Enemas

Here is one for the not-so faint of heart. Did you know that by having an enema done, you are giving your vagus nerve the workout of a lifetime?

It doesn't sound like fun, but your vagus nerve will love you for it! Enemas are somewhat like a marathon or

100 meter dash for your vagus nerve. By expanding your bowel with a coffee enema, you are increasing your vagus nerves activation levels.

This deep (please excuse the pun) cleansing of your insides is accomplished by overall increasing the liver's ability as well as capacity to filter out the toxins in the blood. In the meantime, the liver is also able to cleanse itself of these toxins by releasing bile into the small and large intestines where it is well on its way toward evacuation through your bowels. Your full amount of blood in your body is constantly circulation through your liver at a rapid rate of a full cleanse every three minutes.

When you insert liquid into the rectum, your body must hold it in. This exerts control over your body and activates the pelvis, which also activates the vagus nerve. Resisting the urge to defecate is actually very helpful in toning the vagus nerve, so enemas can be useful for this purpose, but the type of enema is also important.

Coffee can be used to give yourself an enema that will stimulate the vagus nerve. Any liquid will help with this, but coffee is best, because it contains compounds that actually stimulate nerve endings. In addition, it gets the bile ducts flowing, which helps with digestion.

Enemas in general, as well as those with coffee, help flush toxins out of the bowels, too. This reduces inflammation and helps improve vagal tone. You can make your own enema from cool coffee, or you can buy pre-made enemas in bottles that are easily used. If you make your own, stick to one teaspoon of coffee grounds per enema, as it can be too strong to use full coffee.

If you are retaining your coffee enema for up to 15 minutes or longer, the blood in the system is able to circulate through the liver a few times for cleansing and works much like a dialysis treatment would. The water content of the coffee enema will stimulate the gut into a form of intestinal peristalsis in order to help cleanse and empty the large intestine of any accumulated toxins and bile that have been removed from the system.

When you seek to use the vagus nerve through a coffee enema, you are effectively forcing the point of stimulation of the neurons within the guts. Just as how your muscles will atrophy when you cannot use them, your nerves struggle to function after going unused for an extended period of time. They start to lose their ability to function. This is what the coffee enema is addressing—when you are using a coffee enema, you are effectively triggering the nerve pathways within the colon to begin communicating with the vagus nerve and therefore the brain again.

This works primarily because the colon's job is to absorb the liquid that is within your waste—this keeps you from constantly excreting water that your body otherwise needs to stay hydrated. When you use a coffee enema, then, you are triggering the absorption of liquid into your colon. There are two key acids that are present in coffee that are important. These are kahweol and cafestol palmitate. Your colon absorbs these, and as it does so, the acids boost the production of the enzymes in the liver by upwards of 700%.

When you trigger these enzymes, you then trigger a detoxification process—the enzyme produced then binds to any of the toxins within the liver and then excretes the waste. Considering how frequently the body's blood supply circulates through the liver, once every three minutes, you can effectively filter out your blood incredibly quickly.

Through the use of these enemas, you will start to see all sorts of regulation—you will see that bowel function and digestion starts to improve as the nerves are reactivated and strengthened. Of course, if you are sensitive to caffeine, you may be a bit wary about this process. However, the enema process does not cause much of the caffeine to be absorbed in the first place. The body does not naturally absorb caffeine through the colon, and you are likely to absorb 3.5x less caffeine through an enema that you would otherwise ingest drinking the coffee.

Laugh Loud and Laugh Hard

By laughing, your body releases many endorphins into your body that create a natural high. With this, the laughter that you have can also affect your heart rate, your blood pressure, and the way that you breathe, naturally stimulating the vagus nerve and kicking it into gear to start working on high, then gradual dropping back to relaxation.

Laughter also brings about many other movements that we are not consciously aware of doing, such as moving the muscles in our faces, moving our chest, diaphragm, and even your stomach muscles. It's beginning to sound like a good gym workout without the membership card! Find those funny friends and family members and hover with them for a while, or go to see a comedian if you'd like to give your vagus nerve a thorough workout.

Be gentle on yourself though, as laughing a bit too hard has also been known to overstimulate the vagus nerve and can cause sudden fainting, urination, or coughing fits where you end up with the whole family slamming you on the back while you're choking on your own saliva!

This also in turn causes the eyes to tear up. Just another fun part of stimulating your vagus nerve.

Electrical (Direct) Vagus Nerve Stimulation

When treating epilepsy with a vagus nerve stimulator, there are several potential side effects. Some of them are annoying, but tolerable, while others may be incredibly harmful to the individual. One of the side effects listed for the VNS is cardiac death, which of course, is a terrifying thought to face if you are considering this implant for yourself. Beyond that, there are several other side effects listed:

- Bradycardia
- Nausea
- Struggling to swallow
- Changes to the voice
- Hoarseness and coughing
- Shortness of breath
- Discomfort, pain, or tingling
- Headaches
- Sleepiness
- Sleep apneas

For someone seriously considering this treatment, these symptoms and side effects can be enough to entirely forego this treatment altogether. That is, of course, always an option for you. Just because a doctor has recommended one of these devices does not mean that you have to opt to have it implanted. This is not the only way to trigger the vagus nerve either—there are several methods that you can use to naturally trigger the vagus nerve as well.

Singing to Stimulate the Vagus Nerve

The vagus nerve is known to pass from the brainstem past the inner ear as well as the vocal cords, so it is only fitting that humming and singing will also stimulate this nerve and give off a calming effect on the system.

Have you ever wondered why so many people, when they meditate, seem to moan? In fact, if you heard meditation as a concept, was your first thought to think of someone sitting, cross-legged and saying, "OM" in a really deep voice? This is for a good reason—that sort of noise directly stimulates the vagus nerve. While it most likely was not understood at the time how this sort of movement and sound would directly impact the individuals and why these sort of chants and hums would trigger such a state of calm, it has been found to do so.

This is because it triggers the vagus nerve, and as you trigger the vagus nerve, you encourage your body to go into a parasympathetic state instead of allowing the sympathetic responses to rule your body. As you learn to take back that control, learning how to activate your vagus nerve on a whim, you can force yourself into feeling calmer, even if you were in the middle of an anxiety attack just moments earlier.

When you sing, or hum or chant or do anything else that makes sound at the back of your throat, you are using your vocal cords. These cords tie into the vagus nerve—or rather, the vagus nerve ties around them, and as you make these deep, low, guttural sounds, you are actively stimulating your vagus nerve, almost directly. As you do so, you are essentially exercising your vagus nerve, allowing yourself to increase the tone of your nerve, which can then enable you to better regulate yourself.

As you are stimulating the vagus nerve, you activate it, and as you activate it, you create the effect of calming yourself down. Your nerve communicates to your brain that it has been stimulated and therefore it is time for the body to relax and calm down. This is exactly why these sorts of sounds are so frequently used in meditation, yoga, and other forms of movement and mindfulness that are meant to control your ability to calm yourself down.

Further, as you go through this process through humming or singing, you are forcing yourself to manage your breathing. As you do so, you are activating your vagus nerve in yet another way as well. This may not be the most practical of methods, as there are plenty of situations in which singing to yourself is not necessarily going to be welcomed—you cannot just burst into song during your next job interview or while you are stressing out as you walk down the street. Well, you can, but your results will probably not be what you were hoping for!

However, this can be used when you are on your own. If you are awake late at night and struggling to sleep, for example, you may be able to sing to yourself in order to trigger yourself to start to calm down. If you are in your car driving down the freeway and stressed out because you are, you can always try singing as well.

When you want to use these processes to activate your own vagus nerve, you want to think big, low, and guttural. The deeper the sound, the more likely it is that your vocal cord's movements and vibrations will penetrate the vagus nerve, and the more likely it is that your breathing will be regulated properly to get the right effect. This means that if you wish to do so, you can try singing along to a song that you know is lower and throatier, for example, Adele sings plenty of songs that would engage the notes necessary for this process.

When in doubt or when you do not have a song in mind, you can simply hum to yourself. All you need to do is make sure that your note is deep, loud, and consistent. When you do this, do not worry about embarrassing yourself or trying to be perfect—you are not attempting to become a rock star; you are attempting to regulate your vagus nerve, which is entirely unrelated. You do not have to be good to get the desired effects or to ensure that you are comfortable—all you need to do is make sure that you trigger the right part of your anatomy to get the desired result.

Mindfulness to Stimulate the Vagus Nerve

Mindfulness is a process through which you become aware of your body, relaxing deeply and allowing your body to go through its thought processes without interruption or influence. When you go through mindfulness, you are effectively meditating, and doing so can have fantastic results on your mental health. This sort of meditation can directly influence your state of mind, helping to cope with depression and anxiety.

It can make you happier and more able to focus and function. It can help people cope with pain. It has also been shown to reduce the biomarkers for inflammation.

Now, compare those effects of mindfulness to those that you have learned about thus far through learning about the vagus nerve—they are incredibly similar. Thanks to how similar they are, what happens the two are connected together?

The answer is that you get increased results. You are able to remain calm while also getting all of the fantastic benefits of stimulating the vagus nerve in the first place. The best way to do this, then, is to utilize vagus nerve stimulation into your mindfulness routine.

Mindfulness allows for the individual to essentially detach from emotions, pain, or anything else that is actively occurring at that moment that is unpleasant or uncomfortable. This means, then, that the individual can better cope with any discomfort. In coping better, the individual can then manage their ability to relax and cope, effectively ensuring that they are able to regulate their heart rate.

Through breathing techniques during mindfulness, you take control of your physical self. This allows you to take deep breaths and directly impact your vagus nerve and therefore heart rate. Doing so then enables you to better regulate, and that is likely where some of the anti-inflammatory benefits of mindfulness come into play. This will create a compounded effect in which you are able to better trigger the vagus nerve and create a better effect overall.

When you are utilizing mindfulness, you are effectively teaching yourself to pay attention to the moment that you are in right then. You are entirely accepting what is happening around you and because of that, you are able to better regulate your own emotional response. You are willing to accept exactly what is going on, and because of that acceptance, you can then calm yourself down and focus on your breathing. As you do, you find that you are far more capable of coping with whatever is happening around you in the first place. Most often, these techniques go hand-in-hand with coping with stress or anxiety, both of which the vagus nerve can help manage.

In order to begin, start by sitting down somewhere that you know you will be comfortable and where you can remain relatively uninterrupted. Straighten out your back, allow your feet to rest on the floor and place your hands onto your legs. Your arms and shoulders should be relaxed, though your back must remain straight at this point. You can keep your eyes opened or closed, depending on your own comfort. Whatever you prefer is fine, so long as you are not being distracted by the world around you.

Now, take a moment to pull in a deep breath. You should inhale deeply through your nose, feeling the air travel through your body and to your lungs. Make the breath long and slow, preferably five seconds as you do so. Hold it for a moment before exhaling out of your mouth. Make a low, deep hum as you do so—you could do the stereotypical "Om" sound or simply hum to yourself, depending on your comfort. Allow the hum to last another five seconds as you breathe through your mouth. You will repeat this process, preferably for ten to fifteen minutes if you can manage it. At first, even just five minutes may seem like a struggle, and that is okay. This process takes practice.

When you are going through this process, you may notice that your thoughts are wandering. Make a quick note of whatever your thoughts went to and then gently redirect your thoughts back to your breathing and humming. Getting distracted is normal from time to time, especially when you are new to the process in general. Instead of worrying about it, instead just focus on your breathing and how you are feeling with every inhale and exhale.

Try to go through this process relatively regularly—once or twice a day is a fantastic beginning point, especially as you are working to tone your vagus nerve and as the times that you can focus are shorter. These practices should be used as frequently as you may find them useful, or as often as you would like to. When you use these processes, you will find yourself returning to a state of calm or relaxation, and that should be enough of a reinforcement that going through this process should quickly be enjoyable and calming. What is important, especially at first, however, is regularity. You want to do this at least daily, even if only for a few quick moments first thing in the morning. Even a little mindfulness is better than no mindfulness!

Movement to Stimulate the Vagus Nerve

When you are using movement in order to stimulate the vagus nerve, you are effectively teaching your vagus nerve to become more flexible. Yoga in particular has been found to be incredibly effective at increasing your vagal tone, which would then create all of the desired effects that have been discussed thus far in the book. As you are able to better your vagal tone, you should start to notice that your body is more likely to be highly and fully functional, enabling you to start seeing relief.

As you learn to switch between the systems at will, you will find yourself happier, calmer, and likely feeling healthier as well. Remember, each of these movements will stimulate the vagus nerve in some way—they may directly stimulate it or indirectly stimulate it, but the end result is still the same: A more toned nerve that is more capable of handling anything life happens to throw its way.

Security and Self-Love

When you feel safe, your vagal tone improves. The same goes for feeling happy and positive.

Unfortunately, most people don't really like themselves or their bodies. They find it difficult to take a compliment and will put themselves down. They feel guilty and unhappy about things and are often stressed out, feeling that they just aren't good enough.

Feeling positive about your body and loving who you are can also improve your vagal tone. Self-love is one of the biggest changes you can make in your life, with positive results in your health. You'll find that your immune system functions more efficiently when you are happy with yourself.

Security is another big part of being in control of your life and improving vagal tone. If you feel unsafe, you deal with stress and anxiety. It isn't necessary to have a physical threat right there, though. You can feel stressed if you aren't feeling safe in general. And in today's world, it's very difficult to feel safe. There's always something to worry about.

This was one of the more significant issues that I faced after my vagus nerve was damaged. Before the antibiotic ruined my body, I rarely felt anxious or stressed. All that changed after my vagus nerve was damaged. Suddenly, I was dealing with far more anxiety than before. In addition to the pain, I felt panicky every time I had to do anything outside my comfort zone. Then it got worse. I ended up anxious and stressed over the simplest of things. Even picking my children up from school became a difficult situation. My brain raced over all the things that could go wrong at any given moment and I never truly felt safe.

How can you increase your feeling of security? That depends on the person. In some cases, you may need to take physical steps to make yourself feel safer. This could mean you take the time to install locks on your doors, get a guard dog, etc. These will help you feel safer on the outside. However, you also need to feel secure mentally.

Create a space for yourself where you can relax and detox from the stress of everyday life. This should be an area that reduces anxiety and makes you feel happy and loved. Feeling secure can help your vagus nerve increase tone, so it's worth working on this.

Having a high vagal tone also helps with feeling safe, so it's a cycle that only strengthens as you improve it.

Gratitude

Don't underestimate the power of positive thinking on your vagus nerve health. In fact, it has been proven that a grateful attitude is most prevalent in those with high vagal tone. If your vagal tone is high when you're resting, you are more likely to experience pleasant feelings like gratitude, compassion, love, and will be happier than those with low vagal tone.

You can build on this happiness and increase your vagus nerve tone by developing a habit of being grateful. This is like any other habit, where you need to keep building on it regularly. Here are a few ways you can increase your gratitude:

Keep a gratitude journal: Make a point of writing down at least three things every day that you're grateful for. There will be days when you don't feel like anything is worth saying thanks for, but there is always something. It may be a little thing, like being able to get up in the morning or coffee. There's no shortage of things that you can be thankful for. By focusing on these things every single day, you'll eventually start noticing more things to be grateful for and this will only build.

Say thank you every day: People do things for you every day. Even if they are supposed to do it because it's their job, such as a waitress or bank teller, be sure to say thank you. That little bit of gratitude can have a bit impact, not only on your life, but on other people's lives. You can even go a bit further if you want, by leaving a generous tip or even a note.

Be with people you love: You can't help but feel grateful and happy when you are around those you love. Make a point of spending time with those special people. Have some tea together, go for a walk, or just sit and chat. You'll find yourself calmer and happier when you spend time with these people.

Be mindful: It's easy to start going through your day on rote, not really thinking about what you're doing as you do the same things you do every day. It's important to stay present as you complete your daily tasks. You can do this by focusing on what you are doing and finding pleasure in the individual task that you are accomplishing. Even doing the dishes can be an enlightening experience if you focus.

Choose happiness: It's important to decide to be happy. This doesn't always work, of course, because you can feel other emotions and sometimes they are more than overwhelming. However, happiness is often a choice and you need to make that choice every day. When you wake up in the morning, take a moment to think about your life and decide that today, you will be happy.

Your daily attitude will have a lot to do with vagal tone. It's also beneficial to your mental attitude to be happy and calm. If it takes raising your vagal tone to do that, then you can start with the exercises I've shared here to get you started.

Chiropractor

Your body needs to be in good condition in order to release the vagus nerve and tone it. If you have any blockages throughout your body or if you are out of alignment, it can affect the overall tone of the nerve.

A good chiropractor will be able to treat any blockages that the nerve might have and release it. You'll find that it is much easier to tone your nerve when it is unblocked, so a visit to the chiropractor from time to time is a good idea.

Sex

We have a sex drive for a reason and aside from reproductive purposes, sex can be an excellent way to stimulate the vagus nerve. Any activity that engages the pelvis, such as Kegels, can be used to activate your vagus nerve and sex is the ultimate way to engage the pelvis and stimulate the various nerve endings found there.

However, sex isn't just about pleasure and orgasm, though these are very good ways to boost vagal tone. When you engage in intercourse or even just foreplay, with someone, you are engaging in social interaction and a very intimate method of connecting with another human being. This can gives you a double whammy when it comes to vagal tone and can cause you to feel happier and calmer overall.

Of course, this doesn't mean you should engage in sex with anyone. Even self-pleasuring techniques can give you half of the equation and help boost your vagal tone. However, if you have a special someone to enjoy intimate time with, you'll definitely notice the benefits over time.

Acupressure and Acupuncture

Acupuncture and acupressure are very similar, apart from the fact that one uses pressure and the other uses very thin needles to stimulate specific pressure points. Both methods allow you to physically stimulate the vagus nerve and enhance the parasympathetic reaction. It's considered a good alternative to the implant that we looked at previously.

By inserting needles or adding pressure to specific points in the body, it's possible to stimulate the vagus nerve and rapidly improve its tone. This is something you can do at any practitioner's office and they should be well aware of which points to use in order to open up the nerve's function.

Each of these methods can be done easily and will not cause you further harm. If you are serious about activating your vagus nerve, I highly suggest you select three or four of these activities and schedule them into your daily routine. It shouldn't add too much time to your day and the results can be incredible.

Music and Binaural Beats

Certain types of sound can help your brain work better. This has been known for a while now, but there are more and more studies being done on neuroplasticity and music. You may notice that music affects you. It can give you energy or make you feel low-key. Some music is anger-inducing, while other music can calm you. This is all very important to notice, since you can actually make use of the noise to help your vagal tone.

Many people use music as a way to control their moods, but you can take it a step further and add in binaural beats. These are designed to stimulate the brain, but they are also used to tone the vagus nerve.

Binaural beats are two or more similar sine waves. They need to be pure tone and usually work best with earphones, as they are presented in each ear. As an example, a 500 Hz pure tone could be played in one ear, while a 480 Hz pure tone would be in the other ear. The result is an auditory illusion, which increases the neuroplasticity of the brain and makes it more open to memories and studying.

Binaural beats are considered entrainment, where a duo of autonomous rhythmic oscillators work together to interact and synchronize. This technology can be used to affect the body in various ways, including changing your heart rate, relaxation, and blood pressure, among other things. It is also used to boost memory and increase focus.

Regular music is often mixed with binaural beats to make it easier to listen to the odd rhythms. You can listen to the music while the binaural beats work with your brain to stimulate it and to create a higher state of alertness or a more relaxed state. Different beats are used, depending on the desired result. You can use them to help you sleep, to keep you awake without caffeine and even to help regulate your moods and offset depression. They all work with the vagus nerve, so when used in conjunction with the other methods in this book, you'll find entrainment to be particularly effective in building vagal tone.

Even if you don't incorporate binaural beats into your vagal tone routine, you should definitely consider some music. Opt for something that you enjoy and that feels good. You can listen to music on your morning commute to improve your mood and boost tone, or use it whenever you have a short break.

Prayer

Prayer isn't for anyone, but if you pray to someone or something, then this can help tone the vagus nerve, as well. The act of praying is very much like meditation and it can work similarly to meditation in toning the vagus nerve. When you pray, you are completely focused on the prayer. This clears your mind and brings calmness, but it is more than just that.

Having a belief in a more powerful being or force than yourself can give hope and a feeling of security. These are two things that contribute to the wellbeing of your nervous system.

Visualization

Your mind is a powerful part of your body and it isn't used as much as it could be to improve overall health. If you've never heard of visualization and body awareness, now is a great time to start practicing both. This can be done in conjunction with deep breathing and meditation if you like.

Basically, you will close your eyes and visualize or imagine your vagus nerve. Start from the top of the body and imagine it reaching out to your throat. Visualize it helping you inhale and exhale, smoothly and perfectly. Imagine the nerve reaching out to the various organs. You may not be able to actually control these organs, but you can visualize them working perfectly.

You can also focus on your heartbeat and consciously try to slow it if you like. Just being aware of the beating is often enough to activate the vagus nerve, though. Likewise, focus on the digestive system and visualize it working perfectly. This can actually result in better function of the GI tract.

Focusing on your body and how the vagus nerve works throughout it can be very beneficial. Do this regularly for 10 minutes a day and you will see a surprising improvement in organ function. You may not be able to consciously control your organs, but you can certainly affect their function with your mind.

Practice Generosity

Being generous is something that can also help stimulate your vagus nerve. Not only does this give you a nice dose of daily interaction with other people and boost your social quotient, it's also a great way to feel good about yourself.

Generosity can look like anything that involves giving from yourself. You could give a panhandler some change, but it's not necessarily about offering money. Other ways to be generous include:

Giving your time: Help someone out with a chore, sit and talk with a lonely person, or just spend some time with someone. You could volunteer at a retirement home or just chat with a lonely person in the park. Offer your services at a soup kitchen or food bank and you could make a big difference. There are plenty of opportunities to share your time.

Share your food: Do you have some extra snacks? Why not share with someone who needs a boost? You could easily make their day. It's worth bringing a little extra food with you when you are out and about or going to work so you can share. It's amazing how much better the day gets when you give someone a chocolate bar or packet of crackers.

Give a compliment: Even your words can be generous. Try giving out at least five compliments a day. You'll feel great and the people receiving them will feel good, too. Look for opportunities to tell people something nice about themselves. Don't just focus on appearances, either, you can compliment their inner beauty, too and really make them feel great. In some cases, complimenting someone who is always grumpy or in a bad mood can even turn their day around.

Pay for the person behind you: In the drive-through or at a grocery store, pick up the tab for someone else and make their day while boosting your vagal tone. You never know what someone else is going through and you could easily change the course of their day while you're going about your regular routine.

Foster a pet: If you love animals, why not make room in your home for a rescue? You can either adopt the pet or give it a temporary, loving home until it can find its forever home. Pets also have a warming, relaxing effect on people and can give you a lot more than you give them. Who knows, you may even end up with a failed foster, where you keep the animal you were supposed to give back later.

Let someone cut in line: While driving or standing in line, let someone move ahead of you. It literally costs you nothing but a few seconds or a minute, but it is a generous move that will improve both your moods. Instead of fostering rage and frustration, smile, wave that person ahead and increase that vagal tone.

There are little opportunities to be generous all around us. It doesn't have to be a grand gesture, but even little things can help change the course of someone's day, including yours. In addition, you'll get the added benefits for boosting your vagal tone.

Create a Routine

You need to be activating your vagus nerve on a daily basis and the best way to do that is to simply incorporate the methods in these chapters into your daily routine. Make a schedule that includes as many methods of activating the nervous system as possible. First, look at your schedule as it is today. You probably already have a routine, since most people are creatures of habit. So, when you wake up in the morning, you might shower, dress, then have breakfast, brush your teeth and commute to work. Whatever your routine is, you can adjust it to include more opportunities to stimulate vagal tone and boost it.

In our example routine, you can easily change it up and add to the existing activities. For example:

- Shower - instead of taking a regular shower, turn your water to cold and do a little cold exposure. You can also sing or hum while in the shower, to activate the vagus nerve via your throat and vocal cords.
- Get dressed - do some jumping jacks or stretches before you pull on your clothes and you'll get extra benefits. It doesn't have to be a long workout, just a few stretches to get things activated.

- Eat breakfast - Take the time to really appreciate your food and feel gratitude for it. Chew slowly, experience the flavors and textures, and generally make breakfast about truly appreciating what you have. If you have loved ones, this is a good time to make eye contact and engage socially.
- Brush teeth - gargle the rinse water after you brush your teeth and you'll immediately activate the vagus nerve.
- Commute to work - Sing, chant, or hum as you drive in the car. This is a good time to be generous, as well. You can easily let someone merge in front of you and take the time to smile at others as you drive. It doesn't have to be a huge gesture, but even the little things make a difference.

As you can see, it's fairly easy to incorporate these activities into your daily routine. It's just a little bit of adjustment and you immediately turn each activity into something beneficial. Not only are you cleaning your teeth, but you're also toning your vagus nerve. When you associate specific actions with your daily routine, it becomes easier to remember them and to continue using these techniques each day.

You can also make a point of hugging each family member before you leave the house and when you come home, greeting your co-workers with a smile, and being generous to others as you go about your day. Lunch or breaks make a good time for a short meditation session and you can eat with others to increase your social interactions.

Once you've mapped out your day, you'll see that there are plenty of opportunities to boost your vagal tone throughout the day. Doing so consciously will help you start adding more and more specific actions into your routine.

Timing: How Much Stimulation is Needed?

Every single person is different and the amount of damage and the level of vagal tone will vary from person to person. What you need is completely different from what I need.

If you're not sure how much to start with, aim for 20 minutes in the morning and evening. You can incorporate more activities into your daily routine, of course, but there should be roughly 10-20 minutes morning and night of specific vagal toning activities.

Studies with the vagus nerve stimulator showed that it didn't improve vagal tone when the nerve was stimulated constantly. It turned out to be more effective stimulating it just several times a day. Keep this in mind as you go about your daily routine and make sure that you do something to activate your nerve every couple of hours.

It's very important that you set up a routine, because without it, you'll likely forget to do anything and that can only cause you to continue suffering. They say it takes 21 days to create a habit and once you have established a habit, you can continue to do it without even thinking about it.

Decide what you want your habit to be and get started today. The longer you wait, the more you have to deal with ongoing pain and symptoms that could be lessened if you just took action. While it does require time to build vagal tone and repair nerve damage, if you start today, you can look forward to experiencing relief sooner.

Conclusion

This guide was intended to be a guide to learning all about the vagus nerve, how to recognize problems that may arise when the vagus nerve is struggling to function effectively, and then how best to manage any distress that goes along with the vagus nerve malfunction in the first place. As you read through this book, hopefully you found some information that was insightful, beneficial to you, and useful to use.

Within this book, you were introduced to several different concepts, ranging from the vagus nerve even existing to the mind-gut axis, the several systems that the nervous system is responsible for, and more. You were taught several ways that you could activate your vagus nerve at home, some of which were conventional and others a bit less so.

From here, you must choose what you would like to do next. If you are interested in learning more about the biopsychology of the vagus nerve, that is one option for you—you could make it a point to study the interaction between the various nervous systems, learning more about exactly how that one (not-so-) little nerve is able to interact with your entire body, uniting a mind and a body together into one cohesive force.

If you wish to discuss getting a vagus nerve stimulator implanted, you can move forward with discussing that process with your doctor to discover if that is an option for you in the first place. You can see if that is a valid treatment plan, and if it is, you can move forward with the process in order to see if a direct stimulator will aid you in overcoming your pathologies once and for all.

If you wish to take control of your vagus nerve yourself, you can begin some of the techniques discussed within this book.

No matter what, there is no real right answer on where to go from here. The best answer is the one that helps you lessen your own suffering. Whether you are currently suffering from anxiety, arthritis, epilepsy, or any other chronic illness or disorder that is causing you to be unhappy, what matters most is that you can trigger the happiness that you deserve, once and for all. With the help of the vagus nerve, you should be able to achieve that result with ease.

Understanding how your body works and how you can reach your goals in terms of maintaining a healthy body is a great way to tap into the body's potential for self-healing and self-regulation.

Accessing the power of the vagus nerve through stimulation gives you back the power to take charge of your health and ensure that your body is functioning at its best.

You hold in your hands a compendium of knowledge about the vagus nerve, its influence on the body and how you can take care of it. By knowing more about the vagus nerve, you are one step closer to not only being aware of its powerful influences, but also how you can take care of it.

It is now up to you to focus on reducing inflammation in the body, lowering the levels of stress, and using proper routines to improve the conditions of your vagus nerve.

With a plan in place, you will be more than ready to start tapping into the tremendous potential that your vagus nerve has to offer. Are you ready to start seeing results? Follow everything I've shared with you in this book and you will begin to see changes that you never thought were possible.

www.ingramcontent.com/pod-product-compliance
Lightning Source LLC
Chambersburg PA
CBHW072023230526
45466CB00019B/216